The Subtalar Joint

Editor

NORMAN ESPINOSA

FOOT AND ANKLE CLINICS

www.foot.theclinics.com

Consulting Editor
MARK S. MYERSON

September 2018 • Volume 23 • Number 3

ELSEVIER

1600 John F. Kennedy Boulevard • Suite 1800 • Philadelphia, Pennsylvania, 19103-2899

http://www.theclinics.com

FOOT AND ANKLE CLINICS Volume 23, Number 3
September 2018 ISSN 1083-7515, ISBN-13: 978-0-323-58399-2

Editor: Lauren Boyle
Developmental Editor: Meredith Madeira

Foot and Ankle Clinics (ISSN 1083-7515) is published quarterly by Elsevier, Inc., 360 Park Avenue South, New York, NY 10010-1710. Months of issue are March, June, September, and December. Periodicals postage paid at New York, NY, and additional mailing offices. Subscription price per year is $326.00 (US individuals), $519.00 (US institutions), $100.00 (US students), $367.00 (Canadian individuals), $623.00 (Canadian institutions), $215.00 (Canadian students), $460.00 (international individuals), $623.00 (international institutions), and $215.00 (international students). To receive student/resident rate, orders must be accompanied by name of affiliated institution, date of term, and the signature of program/residency coordinator on institution letterhead. Orders will be billed at individual rate until proof of status is received. Foreign air speed delivery is included in all Clinics subscription prices. All prices are subject to change without notice. **POSTMASTER:** Send address changes to Foot and Ankle Clinics, Elsevier Health Sciences Division, Subscription Customer Service, 3251 Riverport Lane, Maryland Heights, MO 63043. **Customer Service: 1-800-654-2452 (US and Canada). From outside of the United States and Canada, call 314-447-8871. Fax: 314-447-8029. E-mail: JournalsCustomerService-usa@ elsevier.com (for print support); JournalsOnlineSupport-usa@elsevier.com (for online support).**

Reprints. For copies of 100 or more, of articles in this publication, please contact the Commercial Reprints Department, Elsevier Inc., 360 Park Avenue South, New York, NY 10010-1710. Tel.: 212-633-3874; Fax: 212-633-3820; E-mail: reprints@elsevier.com.

Contributors

CONSULTING EDITOR

MARK S. MYERSON, MD
Medical Director, The Foot and Ankle Association, Inc, Baltimore, Maryland, USA

EDITOR

NORMAN ESPINOSA, MD
Institute for Foot and Ankle Reconstruction, Foot and Ankle Surgery, FussInstitut Zurich, Zurich, Switzerland

AUTHORS

JAN BARTONÍČEK, MD, DSc
Professor, Departments of Orthopaedics and Anatomy, First Faculty of Medicine, Charles University, Central Military Hospital Prague, Prague, Czech Republic

NORMAN ESPINOSA, MD
Institute for Foot and Ankle Reconstruction, Foot and Ankle Surgery, FussInstitut Zurich, Zurich, Switzerland

LUKAS DANIEL ISELIN, MD
Team Leader, Foot and Ankle Surgery, Department of Orhtopaedic Surgery and Traumatology, Kantonsspital Lucerne, Lucerne, Switzerland

GEORG KLAMMER, MD
Foot and Ankle Surgery, FussInstitut Zurich, Zurich, Switzerland

LYNDON MASON, MB BCh, MRCS (Eng), FRCS (Tr&Orth)
Consultant, Trauma and Orthopaedic Department, Aintree University Hospital, Honorary Senior Clinical Lecturer, Liverpool University, Liverpool, United Kingdom

RODRIGO MELO, MD
Staff Member, Foot and Ankle Unit, Hospital Militar, Universidad de Los Andes, Santiago, Chile

THOMAS MITTLMEIER, MD, PhD
Department of Trauma, Hand and Reconstructive Surgery, Professor and Chairman, Rostock University Medical Center, Rostock, Germany

ANDREW MOLLOY, MB ChB, MRCS (Ed), FRCS (Tr&Orth)
Consultant, Trauma and Orthopaedic Department, Aintree University Hospital, Honorary Senior Clinical Lecturer, Liverpool University, Liverpool, United Kingdom

ONDŘEJ NAŇKA, MD, PhD
Department of Anatomy, First Faculty of Medicine, Charles University Prague, Czech Republic

CRISTIAN A. ORTIZ, MD
Head, Foot and Ankle Department, Clinica Universidad de los Andes, Universidad del, Santiago, Chile

KYEONG-HYEON PARK, MD
Department of Orthopedic Surgery, Kyungpook National University Hospital, Daegu, Korea

STEFAN RAMMELT, MD, PhD
Professor, Head of the Foot and Ankle Section, University Center for Orthopedics and Traumatology, University Hospital "Carl Gustav Carus," TU Dresden, Dresden, Germany

ADAM SANGEORZAN, MD
Resident, Department of Orthopaedics and Sports Medicine, Harborview Medical Center, University of Washington, Seattle, Washington, USA

BRUCE SANGEORZAN, MD
Professor, Department of Orthopaedics and Sports Medicine, Harborview Medical Center, University of Washington, Director, Center for Limb Loss and Mobility, VA Puget Sound Medical Center, Seattle, Washington, USA

CHRISTOPH SOMMER, MD
Departement of Surgery, Kantonsspital Graubünden, Chur, Switzerland

CHRISTIAN TINNER, MD
Departement of Surgery, Kantonsspital Graubünden, Chur, Switzerland

ELENA VACAS, MD
Institute for Foot and Ankle Reconstruction, Zurich, Switzerland; Fellow, University Hospital, Madrid, Spain

ARND F. VIEHÖFER, MD, Dipl. Phys
Consultant Foot and Ankle Surgery, Department of Orthopedics, Balgrist University Hospital, Zürich, Switzerland

EMILIO WAGNER, MD
Staff Member, Foot and Ankle Department, Associate Professor, Clinica Alemana, Universidad del Desarrollo, Santiago, Chile

PABLO WAGNER, MD
Foot and Ankle Department, Clinica Alemana, Universidad del Desarrollo, Santiago, Chile

JAMES WIDNALL, MB ChB, MRCS, FRCS (Tr&Orth)
Specialist Registrar, Trauma and Orthopaedic Department, Aintree University Hospital, Liverpool, United Kingdom

STEPHAN H. WIRTH, MD
Head of Foot and Ankle Surgery, Department of Orthopedics, Balgrist University Hospital, Zürich, Switzerland

STEFAN M. ZIMMERMANN, MD
Consultant Foot and Ankle Surgery, Department of Orthopedics, Balgrist University Hospital, Zürich, Switzerland

Editorial Advisory Board

Contents

talocalcaneal coalitions. Subtalar stiffness results in pathologic kinematics with increased risk of ankle sprains, planovalgus foot deformity, and progressive joint degeneration. Resection of the coalition yields good results. Tissue interposition may reduce the risk of reossification, and concomitant deformity should be addressed in the same surgical setting.

Surgical access to the subtalar joint is required in a plethora of pathologic conditions of the hindfoot. The conventional lateral approach can give excellent access to subtalar joint; however, in hindfoot valgus deformities, there can be unacceptable risks of wound problems and incomplete deformity corrections. The medial approach offers good access to the subtalar joint with an increasing evidence base for its use, especially with double fusions in pes planus deformities. The authors review the current evidence in the use of the medial approach for the subtalar joint.

The subtalar joint plays an important role for the hindfoot when accommodating during gait. Joint degeneration may be caused by posttraumatic, inflammatory, and pathologic biomechanical changes. Once conservative treatment has failed, subtalar fusion should be considered. The indication for surgery is based on thorough clinical and radiographic evaluation. Several techniques for subtalar fusion are published in the literature. This article aims to describe a technique for in situ arthrodesis of the subtalar joint, paying special attention to biomechanical aspects as well as preoperative clinical and radiologic workup.

Arthroscopic subtalar fusion is an excellent approach to subtalar pathologic condition where conservative treatment has failed and a fusion has been indicated. Formal contraindications include excessive malalignment and bone loss. The posterior arthroscopic approach is analyzed in this article, including indications, surgical technique, surgical tips, and complications. Excellent results can be expected, including a shorter time to fusion, and faster rehabilitation, including activities of daily living and sports.

The subtalar joint can be altered in its anatomy and biomechanical behavior. It is important to know how to assess the talar declination angle to assess the deformity at the subtalar joint. Consider a straight posterior approach to the subtalar joint and remain liberal in the use of z-shaped Achilles tendon lengthening. A structural bone graft should be used to elevate the talus. Positioning screws should be used to lock the construct.

FOOT AND ANKLE CLINICS

RELATED INTEREST

Clinics in Podiatric Medicine and Surgery, October 2017 (Vol. 34, No. 4)
Surgical Advances in Ankle Arthritis
Alan Ng, *Editor*
Available at: https://www.podiatric.theclinics.com/

THE CLINICS ARE NOW AVAILABLE ONLINE!
Access your subscription at:
www.theclinics.com

Preface
The Subtalar Joint

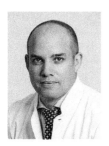

Norman Espinosa, MD
Editor

The subtalar joint is a fascinating structure and, as Leonardo da Vinci would state, "a masterpiece of engineering." The complex structure and its function are not yet completely understood.

This issue of *Foot and Ankle Clinics of North America* provides new insights into the anatomy, biomechanics, and pathologies of the subtalar joint. In addition, this issue provides step-by-step descriptions of various techniques applied to the subtalar joint. Therefore, the reader will receive not only detailed descriptions of how to treat injuries but also solutions regarding the treatment of complex pathologies, including open and arthroscopic approaches.

I have been blessed to find outstanding experts in their fields to contribute to this issue. Every article in it is wonderful and opens the reader to new perspectives. I am sure that it will be of help for many readers, and that it will serve as a cornerstone in the library of many orthopedic foot and ankle surgeons.

Thus, I hope that this issue will stimulate many readers to consider the future and to discover new ideas of how to improve treatment strategies. I would like to thank my collaborators for having made this possible. I also would like to thank Meredith Madeira and Sara Watkins from Elsevier for accompanying me during the evolution of this issue and the publication process.

A special thanks goes to Mark S. Myerson: My mentor and teacher who invited my to design this issue!

Foot Ankle Clin N Am 23 (2018) xi–xii
https://doi.org/10.1016/j.fcl.2018.05.001
1083-7515/18/© 2018 Published by Elsevier Inc.

foot.theclinics.com

Mark is a unique personality and teacher; he taught me most of the secrets of foot and ankle surgery and told me to keep free and to break beyond frontiers. There is always something you can discover!

Norman Espinosa, MD
Institute for Foot and Ankle Reconstruction
Foot and Ankle Surgery
FussInstitut Zurich
Kappelistrasse 7
Zurich 8002, Switzerland

E-mail address:
espinosa@fussinstitut.ch

Anatomy of the Subtalar Joint

Jan Bartoníček, MD, DSc[a,b,]*, Stefan Rammelt, MD, PhD[c], Ondřej Naňka, MD, PhD[b]

KEYWORDS

- Subtalar joint • Spring ligament • Canalis tarsi • Coxa pedis

KEY POINTS

- The subtalar joint may be divided into three separate anatomical parts: the talocalcaneo-navicular joint and the talocalcaneal joint, separated by a conical interosseous tunnel (the canalis and sinus tarsi).
- The talocalcaneonavicular joint may be characterized as a ball-and-socket articulation, also called the coxa pedis.
- The ligaments are an integral part of the coxa pedis, most notably the spring ligament, the medial part of the bifurcate ligament and the dorsal talonavicular ligament. The spring ligament forms a central part of the acetabulum pedis.
- Three-dimensional motion in the subtalar joint complex (eversion/inversion) is guided by the axial alignment of the the talus, calcaneus and navicular, the ligaments, and the shape of the articular surfaces.

INTRODUCTION: GENERAL FEATURES

A description of the talus and its articulation with the surrounding bones (calcaneus, navicular) is highly variable in both the anatomic and clinical literature.[1–22] The anatomic literature distinguishes between individual joints, that is, the talocalcaneonavicular (TCN) and the (posterior) talocalcaneal (TC) joints as 2 separate entities, and uses the term subtalar joint only for the posterior TC articulation (**Fig. 1**). In some textbooks, the subtalar joint complex also includes the calcaneocuboid (CC) joint. Actually, these 3 anatomically separate joints (ie, the TCN, the TC, and the CC) constitute 2 functional units. One of them, called the subtalar joint in the clinical literature, is formed by the TC and TCN joints, allowing a 3-dimensional motion of the

[a] Department of Orthopaedics, First Faculty of Medicine, Charles University, Central Military Hospital Prague, U Vojenské nemocnice 1200, Prague 6, 169 02, Czech Republic; [b] Department of Anatomy, First Faculty of Medicine, Charles University Prague, U Nemocnice 3, Prague 2, 128 00, Czech Republic; [c] University Center of Orthopaedics and Traumatology, University Hospital Carl Gustav Carus, TU Dresden, Fetscherstrasse 74, Dresden 01307, Germany
* Corresponding author. Department of Orthopaedics, First Faculty of Medicine, Charles University, U Vojenské nemocnice 1200, Prague 6, 169 02, Czech Republic.
E-mail address: bartonicek.jan@seznam.cz

Foot Ankle Clin N Am 23 (2018) 315–340
https://doi.org/10.1016/j.fcl.2018.04.001
1083-7515/18/© 2018 Elsevier Inc. All rights reserved.

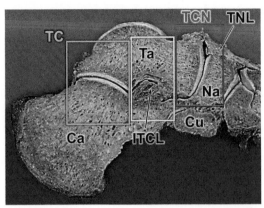

Fig. 1. Sagittal section of the hindfoot. The subtalar joint complex consists of 3 separate anatomic parts: the talocalcaneonavicular joint anteriorly (*red*) and the talocalcaneal joint posteriorly (*green*), separated by the canalis and sinus tarsi (*yellow*). Ca, calcaneus; Cu, cuneiforme; ITCL, interosseous talocalcaneal ligament; Na, navicular; Ta, talus; TC, talocalcaneal joint; TCN, talocalcaneonavicular joint; TNL, talonavicular ligament.

distal foot (lamina pedis or foot plate[13]) in relation to the talus. The other unit, formed by the TN and CC joints and called the transverse tarsal or Chopart joint (articulatio tarsi transversa), is responsible for the motion between the hindfoot (the talus and the calcaneus) and the midfoot (the navicular and the cuboid). Together, the TN, TNC, and CC joints are also termed the triple joint complex because they closely interact with each other.

The subtalar joint may, therefore, be defined from a functional point of view as the osteoligamentous complex formed by 3 bones, that is, the talus, the calcaneus, and the navicular, and the corresponding ligamentous complex. The subtalar joint may be divided into 3 separate anatomic parts: the TCN joint (the anterior part), the TC (the posterior part), separated by a conical interosseous tunnel (the middle part) consisting of the canalis and sinus tarsi (**Fig. 2**). The ligament complex within the latter one is of great importance for the stability and simultaneous action of the TCN and the TC joints.

Function of the subtalar joint complex is determined by the spatial relationship between the talus and the calcaneus. Posteriorly, in the TC joint, the talus is situated directly above the calcaneus, whereas distally the longitudinal axis of the talus deviates by about 35° medially from the lateral aspect of the calcaneus. As a result, the head of the talus lies medial and proximal to the cuboid surface of the calcaneus (**Fig. 3**). This arrangement constitutes the basis of the 2 main columns of the foot, the medial (talar) and the lateral (calcaneal), as well as the medial longitudinal arch of the foot.

The anatomy and function of the subtalar joint have been described in a number of studies.[12–19] The first to publish an anatomic description was Iosiah Weitbrecht (1702–1745) in 1742 (**Fig. 4**).[1] The clinical significance of the TNC joint in the pathomechanics of clubfoot (pes equinovarus) was pointed out by Antonio Scarpa (1752–1832) in 1806, who called the socket of the TNC joint the acetabolo.[2] The subtalar joint evolved from a single joint in early mammals into a complex joint with a more upright axis to adapt the foot to the ground for bipedal gait. Although marsupials still have a single compound inferior articular surface for the talus (the lamina pedis), insectivores and

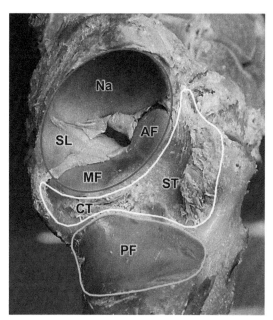

Fig. 2. The 3 components of the subtalar joint marked on the superior aspect of right calcaneus; talocalcaneonavicular joint (*red*), canalis and sinus tarsi (*yellow*), and talocalcaneal joint (*green*). AF, anterior facet; CT, canalis tarsi; MF, middle facet; Na, navicular; PF, posterior facet; SL, spring ligament; ST, sinus tarsi.

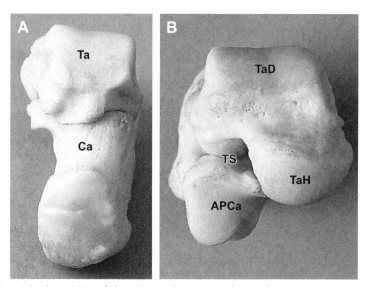

Fig. 3. Spatial relationship of the talus and calcaneus from (*A*) posterior and (*B*) anterior. APCa, anterior process of the calcaneus; Ca, calcaneus; Ta, talus; TaD, talar dome; TaH, talar head; TS, sinus tarsi.

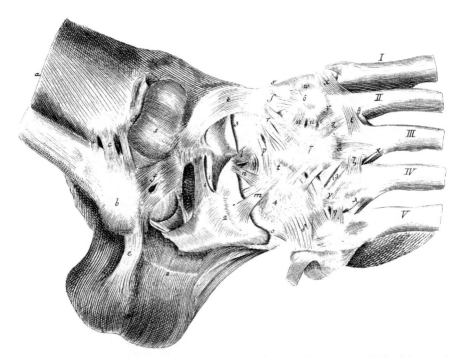

Fig. 4. Ligaments of subtalar joint in the original historical drawing published by Iosiah Weitbrecht in 1742.[1] g, anterior talocalcaneal ligament; ii, cervical ligament; k, talonavicular ligament; l+n, bifurcate ligament (English terminology is used in the legend). (*From* Weitbrecht I. Syndesmologia sive historia ligamentorum corporis humani. Petropoli (Russia): Typographia academiae scientiarum; 1742; with permission.)

primates exhibit a distinctive TC and TCN joint separated by a canalis tarsi with an interosseous ligament.[13]

In the embryonal period in humans, the TC and TCN joints form a single enarthrosis without a clearly visible sinus or canalis tarsi.[16,18] The cartilaginous precursors of the calcaneus and navicular are separated by mesenchymal tissue between the anterior calcaneal process and the navicular.[18] Failure of these bones to completely separate in the fetal period results in calcaneonavicular coalition. The sinus tarsi appears in the 11th week of gestation and the ligaments form develop from mesenchymal precursors beginning with the inferior extensor retinaculum at the 9th week and continuing to the cervical and interosseous ligaments at the 11th to 14th weeks (**Fig. 5**).

TALOCALCANEONAVICULAR JOINT

The TCN joint may be characterized as a ball-and-socket articulation. The resemblance between the hip and TCN joints was mentioned as early as in 1896 by Barclay Smith,[5] who was the first to publish a detailed description of the subtalar joint, valid until today. The term coxa pedis was popularized by Pisani[15,16] in the 1980s. According to Pisani,[15,16] there is not only an anatomic analogy to the hip joint, but also an evolutionary and pathogenetic analogy.

Anatomically, the talar head resembles the femoral head, and the anterior and middle facets of the calcaneus and the talar (posterior) articular surface of the navicular

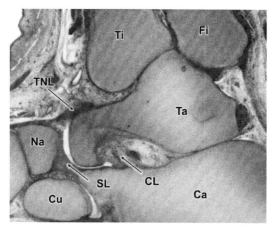

Fig. 5. Ligaments of the subtalar joint on sagittal section in an embryologic specimen at the end of the 13th week of gestation (90 days). Ca, calcaneus; CL, cervical ligament; Cu, cuboid; Fi, fibula; Na, navicular; TNL, talonavicular ligament; SL, spring ligament; Ta, talus; Ti, tibia.

resemble the acetabulum. The 2 bones are connected by a ligamentous complex termed the spring ligament, which forms the central part of the socket. Interestingly, the spring ligament is called the socket ligament (*Pfannenband* in German). From a developmental standpoint, the internal rotation of the femoral head of 40° at birth reciprocates the external rotation of the talar head of 50° at birth. During childhood, both decrease gradually to about 15° at the age of 15 years.[15] Finally, with respect to deformities, Pisani[16] likens the congenital flatfoot deformity (vertical talus) with protrusion of the talar head to the femoral protrusion in coxa profunda and the congenital dislocation of the talus in clubfoot to congenital dislocation of the hip.

Articular Surfaces

The anatomy of the articular facets on the talus and calcaneus is highly variable. Therefore, the articular facets of the calcaneus and talus were classified in various ways by different authors.[14,23–29] This applies not only to the number and shape of the facets, but also to their mutual relationship. It seems that individual variants of articular surfaces are influenced also by the geographic origin of the individuals studied (Europe, Asia, Africa).[23]

Talus

The talar head and neck typically carry 4 articular facets (**Fig. 6**). Two inferior facets, the anterior and middle, articulate with the calcaneus. They may be blended into a single anteromedial facet and even fusions of all articular facets, including the posterior facet at the TC joint obliterating the sinus tarsi, have been described.[20] A triangular inferomedial facet that is situated medially to the anterior calcaneal facet at the talar head articulates with the spring ligament. The largest of all articular surfaces is the convex, ball-shaped distal surface of the head of the talus articulating with the navicular. The fifth, highly inconsistent facet is situated on the anterolateral part of the head of the talus, which articulates with the lateral calcanonavicular ligament (the medial part of the bifurcate ligament).

The middle calcaneal facet is typically larger than the anterior facet, but extensions of both facets have been described.[20] The anterior and middle calcaneal facets are almost flat. The articular facets of the talar head are separated from each other by

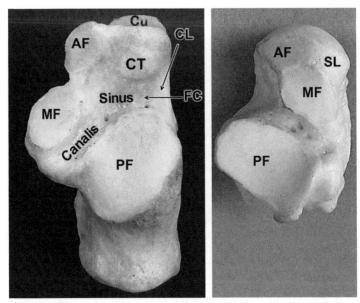

Fig. 6. Articular facets of subtalar joint. AF, anterior facet; Cu, cuboidal facet; CL, crista lateralis; FC, fossa calcanei; MF, middle facet; PF, posterior facet; SL, articular facet for spring ligament.

more or less marked cartilaginous ridges. In rare cases, they are separated by a narrow bony ridge, or the anterior facet is completely absent.[29]

Calcaneus

Two facets on the calcaneus articulate with the head of the talus. The smaller, anterior one is situated on the superior aspect of the anterolateral part of the anterior process of the calcaneus. The larger middle facet covers the superior aspect of the sustentaculum tali. The shape of these facets is as variable as that of their counterparts on the talus and was studied by a number of authors, who classified the individual variants. Bunning and Barnett[23] distinguish between 3 types of articular facets of the calcaneus (**Fig. 7**):

In type A, all 3 facets are distinct structures. The anterior and middle facets are markedly oval shaped, separated by a narrow groove. The posterior facet is separated from the middle facet by the medial part of the calcaneal sulcus, forming the bottom of the tarsal canal. In type B, the anterior and middle facets are either interconnected by a narrow cartilaginous bridge, resulting in the hourglass shape, or the 2 facets blend into a continuous articular surface of an elliptical shape. In type C, all 3 articular facets are fused. The middle and posterior facets are interconnected by a narrow cartilaginous bridge situated close to the medial opening of the tarsal tunnel.

The share of individual types varies considerably in individual studies.[23–28] The incidence of type A ranges between 19% and 67%, with the value of 34% reported most frequently. Similarly, type B ranges between 33% and 78%, with the mean value of 64%. Type C occurs in 1% to 2% of cases.[26] Other, rarer variants have been described in addition to the 3 basic types, such as an absence of the anterior facet.[26] Other variants are tarsal coalitions, most notably TC coalition involving the medial facets and calcaneonavicular coalition.[17]

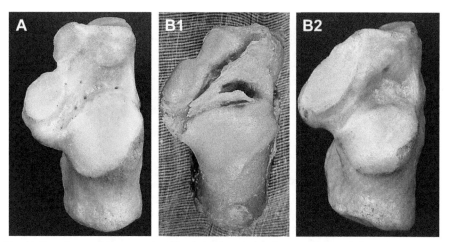

Fig. 7. Bunning and Barnett classification of articular facet variants of the calcaneus. (*A*) Anterior and middle facets are markedly oval shaped, separated by a narrow groove. (*B1*) Anterior and middle facets are either interconnected by a narrow cartilaginous bridge. (*B2*) Anterior and middle facets blend into a continuous elliptical articular facet.

Navicular bone

The facet articulating with the head of the talus has the shape of a horizontal drop. It is concave and is getting flat only toward the plantar aspect.[30–32] In certain cases, this plantar aspect of the navicular projects into a variable bony prominence called the inferior navicular tubercle by Barclay Smith,[5] which has currently been termed as the navicular beak.[32] If present, this beak transforms the articular surface of the navicular into a quadrangular shape.[32]

Ligaments of the Talocalcaneonavicular Joint

The ligaments are an integral part of the coxa pedis, reinforcing the acetabulum, most notably the spring ligament, the medial part of the bifurcate ligament (calcaneonavicular ligament), and the dorsal talonavicular ligament (**Fig. 8**).[14,17,18,33–39]

The spring ligament (inferior or plantar calcaneonavicular ligament) is a ligamentous complex that forms the center of the acetabulum pedis. Its individual parts originate from the anterior edge of the anterior and middle facets of the calcaneus and the sustentaculum tali and insert on the plantar, medial, and dorsal circumference of the navicular. The internal aspect of the spring ligament is partly covered with synovial folds that level out uneven surface between individual parts of the ligament and edges of the adjacent articular surfaces.[18] Barclay Smith[5] described them as "synovial fringes covering pellets of fat."

The individual ligaments constituting the spring ligament have been described and labeled differently in the anatomic literature. Barclay Smith[5] was the first to give a detailed description in 1896. He distinguished between the inferior and superointernal calcaneonavicular ligaments. In 1904, Fick[6] used the term ligamentum acetabuliforme (pars calcaneonaviculare plantare and pars calcaneonaviculare mediale).

The term spring ligament appeared for the first time in the anatomic literature in 1893,[40] based on the studies published by Humphry[41,42] and Hancock.[43,44] In the clinical literature, the term spring ligament or spring ligament complex began to be commonly used in the 1980s. Some authors, however, consider the term spring ligament misleading, based on histologic examination of the ligament[33] or biomechanical analysis.[45]

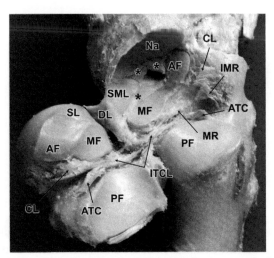

Fig. 8. Right subtalar joint with the talus displaced medially. AF, anterior facet; ATC, anterior talocalcaneal ligament; CL, cervical ligament; DL, deltoid ligament; IMR, intermediate root; ITCL, interosseous talocalcaneal ligament; LR, lateral root; MF, middle facet; MR, medial root (of inferior extensor retinaculum); Na, navicular; PF, posterior facet; SL, articular facet for spring ligament; SML, superomedial ligament. Asterisks, synovial folds.

Recent studies distinguish between 2 parts[32,33] or 3 parts[34,36,37] of the spring ligament. Analysis of these studies shows that it is the varying terminology that poses a problem, rather than description of the whole complex consisting of 3 more or less isolated strands that are clearly discriminable in the plantar and dorsal views (**Figs. 9–11**).

The superomedial ligament (SML), also called the ligamentum neglectum,[46,47] forms the largest, medial part of the spring ligament. Fibers of this rhomboid ligament originate from the edge of the middle facet of the calcaneus and the anteromedial edge of the sustentaculum tali. The fibers originating from the middle facet pass anteromedially and insert on the medial edge of the talar articular surface of the navicular. The fibers originating at the sustentaculum tali run anteriorly and spiral as far as the mediosuperior edge of the articular surface of the navicular. These fibers reinforce the upper edge of the SML and, thus, form the upper edge of the acetabulum pedis resembling by its nature the articular labrum (**Fig. 12**). On the internal aspect of SML there is a triangular or semilunar facet articulating with the corresponding facet on the head of the talus. This facet has a typical shiny fibrocartilaginous surface.[33] Therefore, this part of the SML is called the fibrocartilagonavicularis in the German literature.[6,7,45] The whole SML forms a concave medioplantar articular sling for the head of the talus, having a close relationship with the deltoid ligament and the tibialis posterior tendon. The reinforced upper border of the SML forms the medial labrum of the acetabulum pedis (see **Fig. 9**).

The medial plantar oblique ligament,[37] or the third ligament,[34] forms the middle and thinnest part of the spring ligament.[38] Some authors consider it to be a part of the SML,[33] whereas others consider it a part of the inferior plantar ligament.[32] The medial plantar oblique ligament originates from the anterior edge of the notch between the anterior and middle facets and passes along the lateral border of the SML toward the inferomedial edge of the articular surface of the navicular (see **Figs. 9–11**). It may be separated from the SML by a narrow groove or be almost blended with it.

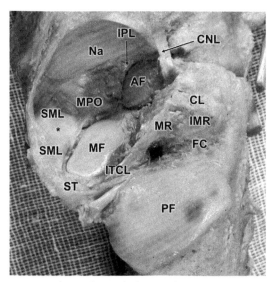

Fig. 9. Spring ligament complex and acetabulum pedis. The 3 distinguishable parts are the superomedial ligament, medial plantar oblique ligament, and inferior plantar ligament (IPL). AF, anterior facet; CL, cervical ligament; CNL, calcaneonavicular dorsal ligament (medial part of bifurcate ligament); FC, fossa calcanei; IMR, intermediate root; IPL, inferior plantar ligament; ITCL, interosseous talocalcanear ligament; MF, middle facet; MPO, medial plantar oblique ligament; MR, medial root; Na, navicular; PF, posterior facet; SML, superomedial ligament; ST, sustentaculum tali. Asterisk, fibrocartilago navicularis.

The inferior plantar ligament (IPL) forms the lateral and the shortest part of the spring ligament. The IPL originates from a small depression (coronoid fossa) on the plantar aspect of the calcaneus between its anterior and medial articulating facets. Fibers of the ligament pass anteriorly and attach to the navicular beak, or, in its absence, to its inferior surface (see **Figs. 8–11**).[32,33]

The spring ligament is 2 to 3 mm thick. Its microscopic structure has been studied by several authors.[14,33,48] Historical studies hypothesized that the ligament consists of elastic fibers.[41–44] Hardy,[48] however, found out in 1951 that "histologically the human plantar calcaneo-navicular ligament consists of dense bundles of collagen fibers, partly parallel in their arrangement but partly interlacing in appearance. In the substance of the ligament no elastic fibers could be detected." Davis[33] has found out that density of the collagen fibers in individual parts of the spring ligament varies and a certain part of the ligament is avascular. The absence of elastic fibers was the reason for questioning the term "spring" ligament.[33,38]

The anterior tibiosubtalar part of the deltoid ligament has a close relationship with the superomedial part of the spring ligament and together they constitute a highly complicated complex that is involved in stabilization of both the ankle and subtalar joints.[49–52] Fibers of the anterior, tibiosubtalar part of the deltoid ligament originate at the anterior colliculus of the medial malleolus, fanning out distally (**Fig. 13**). Posterior fibers insert at the sustentaculum tali. The middle and anterior fibers radiate into the reinforced upper edge of the SML through which the anterior fibers of the deltoid ligament attach to the dorsal aspect of the navicular (**Fig. 14**). This situation resembles the arrangement of the lateral collateral and annular ligaments of the elbow joint. The anterior part of the deltoid ligament has no relation to the talus and inserts on the subtalar structures. The anterior (deep) tibiotalar ligament described by certain

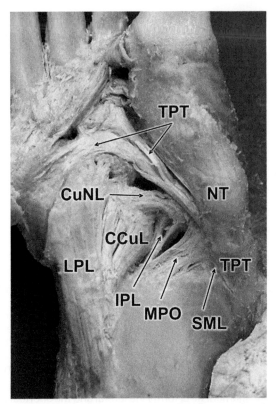

Fig. 10. Plantar aspect of the right talocalcaneonavicular joint. CCuL, calcaneocuboideal ligament; CuNL, cuboideonavicular ligament; IPL, inferior plantar ligament; LPL, long plantar ligament; MPO, medial plantar ligament; NT, navicular tuberosity; SML, superomedial ligament; TPT, tibialis posterior tendon.

authors is actually a part of the joint capsule, which is separated from the deltoid ligament by loose adipose tissue.

The tibialis posterior tendon is intimately connected with the SML. Below the medial malleolus, the tendon turns toward the navicular tuberosity, gets flatter, and passes

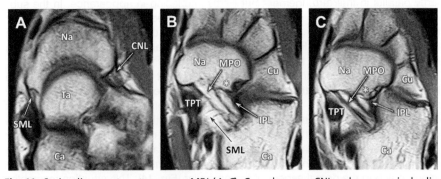

Fig. 11. Spring ligament on transverse MRI (*A–C*). Ca, calcaneus; CNL, calcaneonavicular ligament; Cu, cuboideum; IPL, inferior plantar ligament; MPO, medial plantar oblique ligament; Na, navicular; SML, superomedial ligament; Ta, talar head; TPT, tibialis posterior tendon. Asterisk, navicular beak.

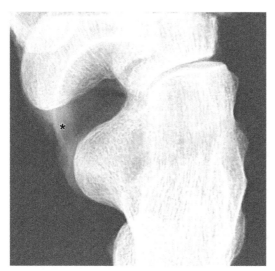

Fig. 12. Radiograph of the acetabulum pedis (anatomic specimen with the talus removed). Asterisk, superomedial ligament.

close to the inferomedial aspect of the SML, gradually acquiring fibrocartilaginous properties (**Fig. 15**). At the navicular tuberosity the tendon divides into 3 parts: medial, central, and lateral (see **Fig. 10**). The strongest, medial part of the tendon inserts into the navicular tuberosity. The central part continues distally and splits into individual

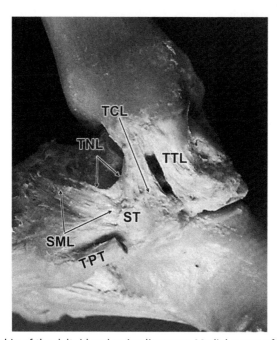

Fig. 13. Relationship of the deltoid and spring ligament. Medial aspect of right ankle. SML, superomedial ligament; ST, sustentaculum tali; TCL, tibiocalcaneal ligament; TNL, tibionavicular ligament; TPT, tibialis posterior tendon; TTL, tibiotalar ligament.

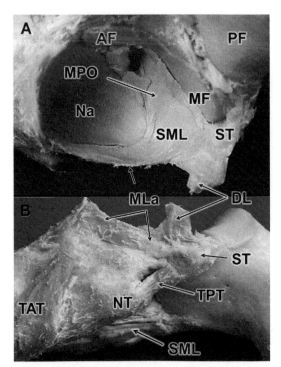

Fig. 14. Right acetabulum pedis from (*A*) superior and (*B*) medial. AF, anterior facet; DL, deltoid ligament; MF, middle facet; MLa "medial labrum" formed by reinforced superior border of SML; MPO, medial plantar ligament; Na, navicular; NT, navicular tuberosity; PF, posterior facet; SML, superomedial ligament; ST, sustentaculum tali; TAT, tibialis anterior tendon; TPT, tibialis posterior tendon.

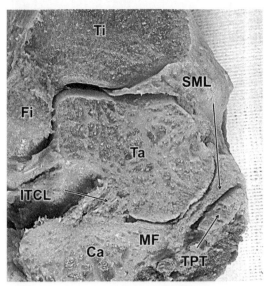

Fig. 15. Relationship of talar head, superomedial ligament and tibialis posterior tendon. Ca, calcaneus; Fi, fibula; ITCL, interosseous talocalcaneal ligament; MF, middle facet; SML, superomedial ligament; Ta, talus; Ti, tibia; TPT, tibialis posterior tendon.

strands inserting at the base of the second to the fifth metatarsal. The short lateral fibers turn laterally in the region of the navicular tuberosity and radiate into the SML.[32]

The bifurcate ligament (Chopart ligament, clavis articulationis Choparti) or the calcaneonaviculocuboidal ligament, is formed by 2 bands contributing to the typical Y or V shape of the ligament.[5,6,38] Their common origin lies on the anteromedial edge of the anterior calcaneal process. The stronger, medial band—the dorsal calcaneonavicular ligament—passes anteromedially, encircles the lateral edge of the anterior facet of the calcaneus, and attaches to the lateral pole of navicular close to the edge of its talar articular surface (**Fig. 16**). The ligament forming the articulating facet on the inferior surface of the talar head completes the lateral labrum of the acetabulum pedis and, at the same time, separates it from the CC joint.

The talonavicular ligament is a broad, trapezoidal, flat ligament reinforcing the posterior portion of the TN joint capsule. The ligament originates from the superior and partly from the lateral aspect of the neck of the talus. Its fibers run anteriorly and medially, slightly converge, and insert on the upper surface of the navicular. Fibers of the deltoid ligament and SML fibers radiate into the medial fibers of the talonavicular ligament (**Fig. 17**). Barclay Smith[5] distinguishes between the superficial, longer, superolateral and the deep, shorter, superomedial portions of the ligament.

CANALIS AND SINUS TARSI

The concave parts of the talus and calcaneus that face each other, primarily the sulcus tali and sulcus calcanei, define a conical interosseous cavity that may be divided into 2 parts (**Fig. 18**). The posteromedial, narrow part is called the canalis tarsi, and the widening, anterolateral part is called the sinus tarsi. The long axis of the canalis and sinus tarsi is oriented anterolaterally at an angle of 45% to the lateral wall of calcaneus.[53]

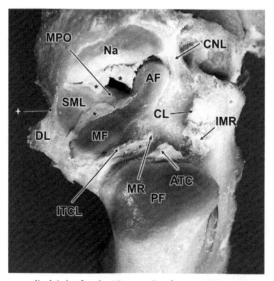

Fig. 16. Acetabulum pedis (*right foot*). AF, anterior facet; ATC, anterior talocalcaneal ligament; CL, cervical ligament; CNL, calcaneonavicular dorsal ligament (medial part of the bifurcate ligament); ITCL, interosseous talocalcanear ligament; MF, middle facet; MPO, medial plantar oblique ligament; MR, medial root and IMR, intermediate root of the inferior extensor retinaculum; Na, navicular; PF, posterior facet; SML, superomedial ligament; white asterisk, tibionavicular part of deltoid ligament. Asterisks, synovial folds.

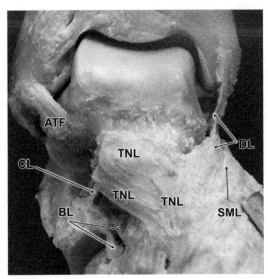

Fig. 17. Dorsal aspect of the right talocalcaneonavicular joint. ATF, anterior talofibular ligament; BL, bifurcate ligament; CL, cervical ligament; DL, deltoid ligament; SML, superomedial ligament; TNL, talonavicular ligament.

The canalis tarsi is anteriorly bound by the middle facets of the talus and the calcaneus; on the posterior side by the posterior facets of the talus and the calcaneus. The sinus tarsi borders on the anterior facets of the talus and calcaneus, the lateral talar process, the lateral wall of the talar neck, the superior edge of the anterior process of the calcaneus and its reinforced lateral crest (crista lateralis).[54] The floor of the sinus

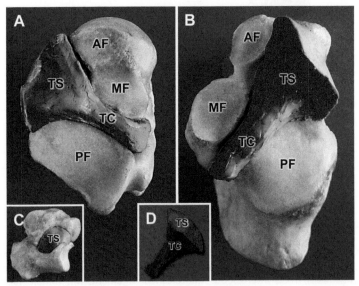

Fig. 18. Anatomy of the tarsal canal and sinus tarsi. (*A*) Plantar view. (*B*) Superior view. (*C*) Anterolateral view. (*D*) Plastic model. AF, anterior facet; MF, middle facet; PF, posterior facet; TC, tarsal canal; TS, sinus tarsi.

tarsi is elevated in the anterolateral part to form a small bony tubercle called the supra-calcaneal tubercle,[54] tuberculus cervicis,[55,56] or cervical tubercle.[54] It gives rise to the cervical ligament. The depressed area of the floor of the sinus tarsi confined by this tubercle, the edge of the posterior talar facet and the lateral crest forms the calcaneal fossa[54] to which the intermediate root of the inferior extensor retinaculum is attached.

The canalis and sinus tarsi contain a complex system of ligaments, the arteries of the canalis and sinus tarsi including anastomoses between them, and fine nerve fibers from the tibial nerve, and the deep and superficial peroneal nerves.[57] The extensor digitorum brevis attaches at the anterolateral edge of the anterior calcaneal process.

Ligamentous System in the Canalis and Sinus Tarsi

The ligaments occupying the canalis and sinus tarsi have been investigated in a number of anatomic studies.[58–65] The sometimes confusing terminology used by individual authors reflects the difficulties when attempting to exactly describe and distinguish this highly complex and variable ligamentous system. The footprint of the ligaments in the canalis and sinus tarsi at the calcaneal insertion is V-shaped (**Figs. 19 and 20**). The following 4 basic structures may be identified regularly in this system: (1) the roots of inferior extensor retinaculum, (2) the cervical ligament, (3) the interosseous TC ligament (ITCL), and (4) the anterior TC ligament (see **Fig. 20**).

The inferior extensor retinaculum is a reinforced part of the fascia of the ankle and foot (**Fig. 21**). It is typically Y-shaped and inserts on the calcaneus through 3 roots described for the first time by Retzius[58] in 1841, and later almost identically by other authors.[5,58,60,64,65]

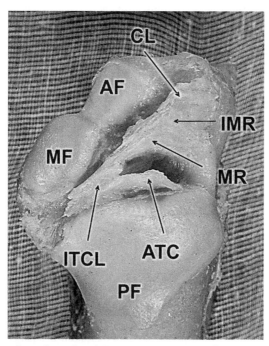

Fig. 19. Ligaments of tarsal canal and sinus tarsi. AF, anterior facet; ATC, anterior talocalcaneal ligament; CL, cervical ligament; IMR, intermediate root of the inferior extensor retinaculum; ITCL, interosseous talocalcaneal ligament; MF, middle facet; MR, medial root; PF, posterior facet.

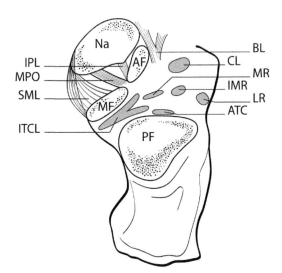

Fig. 20. Ligament footprints of the subtalar joint at the calcaneus. AF, anterior facet; ATC, anterior talocalcaneal ligament; BL, bifurcate ligament; CL, cervical ligament; IMR, intermediate root; IPL, inferior plantar ligament; ITCL, interosseous talocalcaneal ligament; LR, lateral root; MF, middle facet; MPO, medial plantar oblique ligament; MR, medial root; Na, navicular; PF, posterior facet; SML, superomedial ligament.

The stem of the Y of the inferior extensor retinaculum is situated laterally and consists of 2 laminae. The superficial lamina originates at the edge of the sinus tarsi through its lateral root and then passes anteromedially, winding around the extensor digitorum longus tendons. Medially, the retinaculum bifurcates, with 1 limb running toward the medial malleolus and the other toward the navicular tuberosity. The deeper

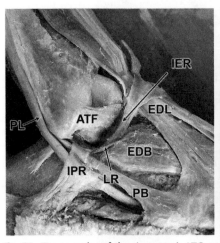
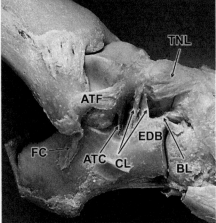

Fig. 21. Topography of the sinus tarsi. ATC, anterior talocalcaneal ligament; ATF, anterior talofibular ligament; BL, bifurcate ligament; CL, cervical ligament; EDB, extensor digitorum brevis; EDL, extensor digitorum longus; FC, fibulocalcaneal ligament; IER, inferior extensor ligament; IPR, inferior peroneal retinaculum; LR, lateral root; PL, peroneus longus; PB, peroneus brevis.

fibers of the lateral stem turn back laterally at the medial aspect of the extensor dig-itorum longus tendons, forming a loop around these tendons and descend into the si-nus tarsi. Thus, they form the deep lamina,[53] inserting at the calcaneus through its intermediate and medial roots. Because of this shape with a loop around the extensor tendons, the inferior extensor retinaculum has also been called the fundiform ligament (sling ligament).[58]

The lateral root of the inferior extensor retinaculum originates from the superficial lamina and attaches to the lateral aspect of the calcaneus directly behind the attach-ment of the extensor digitorum brevis muscle and partly blending with its fascia. The distal fibers of the lateral root blend with the inferior peroneal retinaculum at the ante-rolateral aspect of the calcaneus. The intermediate root originates from the deep lam-ina and inserts at the calcaneal floor of the sinus tarsi medially to the lateral root, close to the lateral crest and posterior to the attachment of the cervical ligament. The medial root is a complex and highly variable structure originating from the deep lamina of the inferior extensor retinaculum.[60,64,65] The fibers of the medial root insert directly behind the cervical ligament. Li and coworkers[65] described a thin lateral component and a broad medial component. In 60% of cases, the medial fibers of the medial root inter-digitate with the fibers of the ITCL.[59,65] The lateral fibers of the medial root blend with the fibers of intermediate root. Unlike the lateral and intermediate roots, certain fibers of the medial root insert on the talar roof of the tarsal canal (**Fig. 22**).[53,59,64] In rare cases, the medial root may be absent.[60]

The cervical ligament[53] or ligamentum talocalcaneum obliquum[60] is a strong extra-articular quadrangular ligament situated in the anterolateral part of the sinus tarsi (see **Fig. 20**; **Figs. 23** and **24**). The term ligamentum cervicis was introduced by Wood Jones in 1944[55] because it connects the neck of the talus and the calcaneus. It inserts on the floor of the sinus tarsi on a small bony prominence, the so-called cervical tuber-cle (see **Fig. 6**). The fibers of the ligament have an oblique course of about 45°, hence, the term oblique TC ligament (lig. talocalcaneum obliquum). They are covered by the

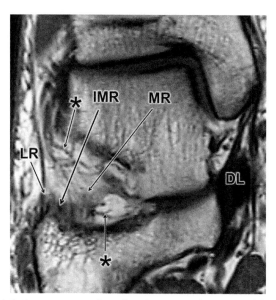

Fig. 22. Roots of inferior extensor retinaculum in a coronal MRI. DL, deltoid ligament; IMR, intermediate root; medial root; LR, lateral root. Asterisks, vessels in the sinus tarsi.

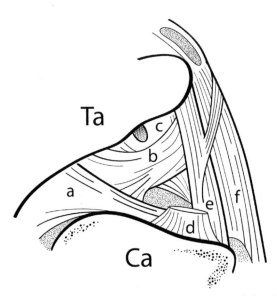

Fig. 23. Ligaments of tarsal canal and sinus tarsi. Posterior view of the right side with the posterior half of the talar dome removed. Ca, calcaneus; Ta, talus. a, talocalcaneal ligament, b, medial root; c, cervical ligament; d, anterior talocalcaneal ligament; e, intermediate root; f, lateral root of the inferior extensor retinaculum. (*Adapted from* Schmidt HM. Gestalt und Befestigung der Bandsysteme in Sinus und Canalis tarsi des Menschen. Acta Anat 1978;102:184–94.)

attachment of the extensor digitorum brevis muscle and the lateral root of the inferior extensor retinaculum (see **Fig. 21**). The ligament typically consists of a single fascicle but in about 20% of cases,[62] it is split into 2 fascicles (see **Fig. 21**). The fibers of the cervical ligament are always crossed.[65] It represents the strongest connection between the talus and calcaneus.

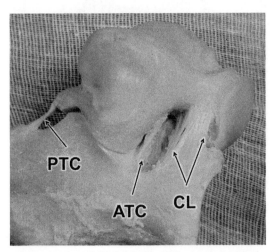

Fig. 24. Ligaments of the sinus tarsi (*right foot*). ATC, anterior talocalcaneal ligament; CL, cervical ligament; PTC, posterior talocalcaneal ligament.

The ITCL occupies the canalis tarsi (see **Figs. 20** and **23**). Therefore, some authors use the term ligament of the tarsal canal (lig. canalis tarsi).[53,59,60] In about 80% of cases,[60,62] fibers of this flat ligament originate in the form of 2 lamellae, the anterior and the posterior, from the talar sulcus and run inferolaterally to the calcaneal sulcus of the tarsal canal at an angle of 35° in the coronal plane.[62] It, therefore, has a V shape in most cases.[60,65] Jotoku and colleagues[64] distinguishes between 3 types of the ligament: the band (93%), the fan (5%), and the multiple (3%) types. In the middle part of the sinus tarsi, the lateral fibers intersect with the medial root of inferior extensor retinaculum. Li and associates[65] found a separate tarsal canal ligament in 62% of 32 specimens. It runs vertically on the medial side of the tarsal canal between the middle TC facet at the sustentaculum and the medial root of the inferior extensor retinaculum.

The anterior TC ligament is considered by some authors as a part of ITCL,[60] whereas according to other investigators,[6,19,64] the ligament is a separate structure reinforcing the anterior portion of the TC joint capsule. It has, therefore, been named the anterior capsular ligament.[20,64,65] This flat ligament originates from the anterior edge of the posterior facet of the talus. Its fibers extend vertically and insert directly in front of the anterior edge of the posterior facet of the calcaneus (see **Figs. 21** and **24**). Its posterior surface is covered by a synovial membrane. Jotoku and associates[64] found this ligament in 95% of 40 specimens. The ligament was always clearly separated from ITCL by adipose tissue.

Vessels and Nerves of the Canalis and Sinus Tarsi

In addition to ligamentous structures, the canalis and sinus tarsi also contain 2 major arteries, the artery of the tarsal canal and the artery of the sinus tarsi.[57,66]

The artery of the tarsal canal (a. canalis tarsi) is typically a branch of the medial plantar artery, and less frequently of the posterior tibial artery. It enters the canalis tarsi through an oval opening between the anterior (tibiosubtalar) and the posterior (tibiotalar) parts of deltoid ligament, located posterior and superior to the sustentaculum tali (see **Fig. 13**). In the canalis tarsi, the artery passes along its talar roof and gives off nutrient intraosseous branches primarily for the talar dome and less for the calcaneus.[66]

The artery of the sinus tarsi (a. sinus tarsi) typically originates from an anastomosis of several arteries, including the lateral tarsal artery, the perforating branch of the peroneal artery, and the anterior lateral malleolar artery. In about 17% of cases, the artery of the sinus tarsi originates directly from the anterior tibial artery. In the sinus tarsi, it splits into a superior and inferior branch. The superior branch extends along the sulcus tali, gives off intraosseous branches for talar dome and anastomoses with the artery of tarsal canal.[57]

The nerve supply of the ligamentous structures in the canalis and sinus tarsi has been described by a number of authors presenting different opinions on their distribution. Numerous Golgi-Mazzoni corpuscles were found in the sinus tarsi and considerably fewer Pacini corpuscles.[15] Viladot and coworkers[14] found nerve endings and Pacinian corpuscles at the periphery of the tarsal canal and the sinus tarsi. There is consensus that the nerve endings on the medial aspect of the sinus tarsi originate from the tibial nerve, and those on the lateral aspect from the deep peroneal nerves.[67] A similar innervation can be seen in the TCN and TC joints.[67]

TALOCALCANEAL JOINT

The TC joint forms the posterior part of the subtalar joint. The talus and calcaneus articulate here through large oval and curved facets. The posterior articular facet of the talus forms the inferior aspect of the body of the talus. It is oval and biconcave, that is, both in the coronal and sagittal planes (see **Figs. 6** and **8**). The posterior facet of the calcaneus has a complementary biconvex shape. Fick[6] defines it as a rounded quadrangle. It forms the upper surface of the central part of the calcaneus, called the thalamus. Some authors provide a different description of the curvature (ie, cylindrical, helicoid, or spiral) and the relationship between the posterior articular facets of the talus and the calcaneus.[6,7,10,20,28,60]

The thin joint capsule inserts close along the circumference of both facets. It is reinforced by several capsular ligaments that are either its part or are close to it.[6,19,61,68,69]

The anterior TC ligament was described in detail elsewhere in this article; it inserts at the posterior border of the sinus tarsi. It is a reinforced portion of the capsule, forming a flat vertical band (see **Fig. 24**).[6,19]

The posterior TC ligament is a flat, short, quadrilateral ligament originating from the posterior tubercle of the posterior process of the talus (see **Fig. 24**; **Figs. 25** and **26**). In certain cases, it originates from the medial tubercle and then it has the shape of a loop winding around the flexor hallucis longus tendon passing in the groove of the same name. The ligament extends posteriorly and inserts on the upper surface of the posterior part of the calcaneus. The ligament is absent in 15% of cases.[6,68]

The lateral TC ligament is a flat, narrow ligament originating from the anterior edge of the apex of the lateral process of the talus. It first passes parallel to the anterior talofibular ligament and then turns toward the distal attachment of the calcaneofibular ligament, where it inserts on the lateral aspect of the calcaneus just medial to this ligament. These 2 ligaments form a horizontal Y-shaped structure (see **Fig. 25**). The lateral TC ligament limits adduction in subtalar joint is variable in terms of its incidence and is reported to be absent in 23% to 50% of cases.[6,20,68] If missing, its function is substituted by the calcaneofibular ligament.

The medial TC ligament has been neglected by a number of authors. The main reason may be the fact that this ligament is overlapped by the complex of the deltoid ligament. The medial TC ligament is a short, flat ligament passing close to the bones, which is present in 54% of cases.[68] The fibers of the ligament originate on the medial surface of the medial tubercle of talus, extend anteriorly and slightly plantarward (inferiorly), and insert on the posterior edge of the sustentaculum tali (see **Fig. 26**).[6,19,20,61,68]

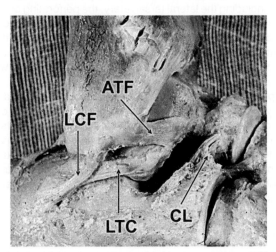

Fig. 25. Lateral talocalcaneal ligament (*right foot*). ATF, anterior talofibular ligament; CL, cervical ligament; LCF, lateral calcaneofibular ligament; LTC, lateral talocalcaneal ligament.

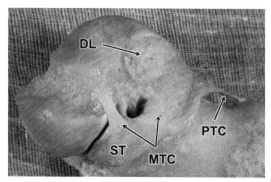

Fig. 26. Medial talocalcaneal ligament (*right foot*). DL, deltoid ligament; MTC, medial talocalcaneal ligament; PTC, posterior talocalcaneal ligament; ST, sustentaculum tali.

In several specimens, we have found another ligament connecting the medial surface of the talus and the calcaneus, which passed close anterior to the medial opening of the canalis tarsi. This finding was fully consistent with a drawing published in 1928 in the anatomic atlas published by Toldt and Hochstetter.[70] Fibers of this ligament extend distally and slightly posteriorly and insert on the sustentaculum tali close to the posterior edge of the medial facet for the talus. In these cases, the medial TC ligament is formed by an anterior and posterior arm, having a V shape and forming the medial opening of canalis tarsi (see **Fig. 26**).

FUNCTION FOLLOWS FORM: IMPLICATIONS ON SUBTALAR JOINT BIOMECHANICS

The complex shape of the subtalar joint with the diverging axes of the talus and calcaneus, the irregular contour of their articular facets, and the ligaments described herein guides a complex motion in the subtalar joint complex. Biomechanics of the subtalar joint have been studied for more than 150 years and the results of these investigations differ considerably among individual authors.[4,6,7,10,16,22,56,71–76] This is addressed in more detail in Adam Sangeorzan and Bruce Sangeorzan's article, "Subtalar Joint Biomechanics: From Normal to Pathologic," in this issue.

The axis of the motion of the subtalar joint is a subject of continuous debate. According to older studies, subtalar motion takes place around a single axis (Henke axis), passing from the lateral aspect of the posterior edge of the calcaneus upward, anteriorly and medially toward the center of the talar head and the navicular at an angle of about 42° to the horizontal plane and 16° to 23° to the sagittal plane.[4,6,7,71,77] According to more recent studies, there is a bundle of axes of movement, depending on the phase of movement in the irregularly shaped subtalar joint.[22,73,78] As nicely illustrated out by MacConaill and Basmajan,[79] relative motion between the talus and calcaneus also depends on which part is fixed and which is moving. The motion generated by a male (calcaneal) ovoid surface moving on a female (talar) surface is that of slide, roll, and spin with the roll in the opposite direction of the slide. If the female ovoid surface moves on the male surface (ie, the talus on the fixed calcaneus), the roll is in the same direction as the slide.[79] The talus and calcaneus move in opposite directions, and the posterior joint surfaces slide on each other. The TC interosseous ligament acts as a pivot for subtalar motion with the center of motion being located in the innermost part of the canalis tarsi.[20] Due this fact and the sometimes V-shaped appearance, the interosseous ligament has been likened to the cruciate ligaments.

Owing to the oblique orientation of the subtalar joint axis, the foot plate exerts a 3-dimensional movement beneath the talus that is best described as inversion (raising the inner margin) and eversion (raising the outer margin) of the foot. The 3 components of inversion are flexion, supination, and adduction; eversion consists of extension (dorsiflexion), pronation, and abduction. Manter[71] recognized a helical (spiral) component to subtalar motion owing to the surface of the posterior calcaneal facet with a helix angle of 12°. Zographos and colleagues[73] states that "The subtalar joint appears to work as a pivot joint during inversion and as a plane joint during eversion." Bony stability in the subtalar joint is greatest in eversion when there is maximum contact and near congruous fit at the posterior TC joint.[20] Inversion and eversion of the foot take place simultaneously in both parts of the subtalar joint, that is, in the TCN and TC joints.

The talus, which has no muscle attachments, behaves as an intercalary bone between the tibiofibular mortis (ankle) and foot plate (subtalar joints), which is controlled by the movement of the surrounding bones. Because of the interaction with the ankle joint, the subtalar joint complex is also called the lower ankle joint (*unteres Sprunggelenk* in the German literature). Ligaments in the canalis and sinus tarsi are of substantial importance for both the stability of the joint during motion and its range. The cervical ligament limits inversion,[14] whereas the ITCL and deltoid ligament limit eversion. The function of ligaments is, therefore, sometimes compared with the function of the cruciate ligaments.[18] The individual range of motion is highly variable with a mean of about 36°.[6,7,71,73,75]

The subtalar joint also closely interacts with the Chopart (midtarsal) joint, most notably through the talonavicular joint, which is also part of both joint complexes. Together they form the triple joint complex. The functional interaction of the longitudinal subtalar and the transverse Chopart joints, is still not completely understood. An understanding of the interaction of these joints and the ankle is essential for understanding of the function of the foot under both normal and pathologic conditions.

SUMMARY

The subtalar joint complex may be divided into 3 separate anatomic parts: the TCN and the TC joints, separated by a conical interosseous tunnel called the canalis and sinus tarsi. The TCN joint may be characterized as a ball-and-socket articulation (coxa pedis). An important part of the coxa pedis is the spring ligament complex formed by 3 parts—the superomedial, medial plantar oblique, and inferior plantar ligaments. The canalis and sinus tarsi, forming the middle part of the subtalar joint, are occupied by roots of the inferior extensor retinaculum, cervical ligament, ITCL, and anterior TC ligament. The capsule of the TC joint is reinforced by relatively constant ligaments. The posterior facet of the talus is biconcave, that of the calcaneus biconvex. Three-dimensional motion in the subtalar joint complex (eversion/inversion) is guided by the axial alignment of the talus, calcaneus and navicular, the ligaments, and the shape of the articular surfaces.

REFERENCES

1. Weitbrecht I. Syndesmologia sive historia ligamentorum corporis humani. Petropoli (Russia): Typographia academiae scientiarum; 1742.
2. Scarpa A. Memoria chirurgica sui piedi torti congeniti dei fanciulli e sulla maniera di correggere questa deformità. Pavia (Italy): Apresso Giusepe Comino; 1806. Available at: https://archive.org/ stream/memoriachirurgi00scargoog#page/n97/ mode/2up.
3. Henle J. Handbuch der Bandlehre des Meschen. Braunschweig (Germany): Fridrich Vieweg und Sohn; 1856.

4. Henke W. Handbuch der Anatomie und Mechanik der Gelenke. Leipzig (Germany): CF Winterʹsche Verhandlung; 1863.
5. Barclay Smith E. The astragalo-calcaneo-navicular joint. J Anat Physiol 1896;30: 390–412.
6. Fick R. Handbuch der Anatomie und Mechanik der Gelenke. Jena (Germany): Fischer; 1904.
7. von Lanz T, Wachsmuth W. Praktische Anatomie. Berlin (Germany): Bein und Statik, Springer; 1938.
8. Testut L, Latarjet A. Traité d'anatomie humaine. Tome premier. Paris (France): Doin et Cie; 1948.
9. Paturet G. Traité d'anatomie humaine. Tome II. Membres supérieur et inférieur. Paris (France): Masson; 1951.
10. Lapidus PW. Subtalar joint, its anatomy and mechanics. Bull Hosp Joint Dis 1955; 16:179–95.
11. Johnston TB, Davis DV, Davis F, editors. Gray's anatomy. 32nd edition. London: Longmans; 1958.
12. Lockhart RD, Hamilton GF, Fyfe FW. Anatomy of the human body. Philadelphia: Lippincott; 1959.
13. Lewis OJ. The joints of the evolving foot. Part II. The intrinsic joints. J Anat 1980; 130:833–57.
14. Viladot A, Lorenzo JC, Salazar J, et al. The subtalar joint: embryology and morphology. Foot Ankle 1984;5:54–66.
15. Pisani G. Trattato di chirurgia del piede. Patologia ortopedica. 2nd edition. Torino (Italy): Edizioni Minerva Medica; 1993.
16. Pisani G. The coxa pedis. Eur J Foot Ankle 1994;1:67–74.
17. Epeldegui T, Delgado E. Acetabulum pedis. Part I: talocalcaneonavicular joint socket in normal foot. J Pediatr Orthop B 1995;4:1–10.
18. de Palma L, Santucci A, Ventura A, et al. Anatomy and embryology of the talocalcaneal joint. Foot Ankle Surg 2003;9:7–18.
19. Linklater J, Hayter CL, Vu D, et al. Anatomy of the subtalar joint and imaging of talo-calcaneal coalition. Skeletal Radiol 2009;38:437–49.
20. Kelikian AS, editor. Sarrafianʹs anatomy of the foot and ankle. 3rd edition. Philadelphia: Lippincott Williams and Wilkins; 2011.
21. Mueller F, Hoechel S, Klaws J, et al. The subtalar and talonavicular joints: a way to access the long-term load intake using conventional CT–data. Surg Radiol Anat 2014;36:463–72.
22. Zwipp H, Rammelt S. Tscherne Unfallchirurgie – Fuss. Berlin (Germany): Springer; 2014.
23. Bunning PSC, Barnett CH. A comparison of adult and foetal talocalcaneal articulations. J Anat 1965;99:71–82.
24. Gupta SC, Gupta CD, Arora AK. Pattern of talar articular facets in Indian calcanei. J Anat 1977;124:651–5.
25. Padmanabhan R. The talar facets of the calcaneus. An anatomical note. Anat Anz 1986;161:389–93.
26. Shahabhour M, Devillé A, Van Roy P, et al. Magnetic resonance imaging of anatomical variants of the subtalar joint. Surg Radiol Anat 2011;33:623–30.
27. Sharada R, Sneha K, Gupta C, et al. Non-metrical study of the pattern of talar articular facets in south Indian dry calcanei. Surg Radiol Anat 2012;34:487–91.
28. Jung MH, Choi BY, Lee JY, et al. Types of subtalar joint facets. Surg Radiol Anat 2015;37:629–38.

29. Nozaki S, Watanabe K, Katayose M. Three-dimensional morphometric analysis of the talus: implication for variations in kinematics of the subtalar joint. Surg Radiol Anat 2017;39(10):1097–106.

30. Schmidt HM. Die Artikulationsflächen der menschlichen Sprunggelenke. Advances in Anatomy and Cell Biology 66. Berlin (Germany): Springer; 1980.

31. Schmidt HM. The plantar ligament of the human proximal tarsus. Folia Morph (Prague) 1980;28:159–61.

32. Golano P, Farinas O, Saenz I. The anatomy of the navicular and periarticular structures. Foot Ankle Clin 2004;9:1–23.

33. Davis WH, Sobel M, DiCarlo EF, et al. Gross, histological, and microvascular anatomy and biomechanical testing of the spring ligament complex. Foot Ankle 1996; 17:95–102.

34. Taniguchi A, Tanaka Y, Takakura Y, et al. Anatomy of the spring ligament. J Bone Joint Surg Am 2003;85-A:2174–8.

35. Rule J, Yao L, Seeger LL. Spring ligament of the ankle: normal MR anatomy. AJR Am J Roentgenol 1993;161:1241–4.

36. Mengiardi B, Zanetti M, Schottle PB, et al. Spring ligament complex: MR imaging-anatomic correlation and findings in asymptomatic subjects. Radiology 2005; 237:242–9.

37. Patil V, Ebraheim NA, Frogameni A, et al. Morphometric dimensions of the calcaneonavicular (Spring) ligament. Foot Ankle Int 2007;28:927–32.

38. Melăo L, Canella C, Weber M, et al. Ligaments of the transverse tarsal joint complex: MRI-Anatomic correlation in cadavers. AJR Am J Roentgenol 2009;193: 662–71.

39. Postan D, Carabelli GS, Poitevin LA. Spring ligament and sustentaculum tali anatomical variations: anatomical research oriented to acquired flat foot study. Foot Ankle Online J 2011;4:1–5.

40. Gray H. Anatomy descriptive and surgical. In: Pick TP, editor. 13th American edition. Philadelphia: Lea Brothers; 1893.

41. Humphry GM. A treatise on the human skeleton. Cambridge (England): Macmillan; 1858.

42. Humphry GM. The human foot and the human hand. Cambridge (England): Macmillan; 1861.

43. Hancock H. Anatomy and surgery of the human foot. Lancet 1866;87/2232: 617–9.

44. Hancock H. A course of lectures on the operative surgery of the foot and ankle-joint. London: Churchill; 1873.

45. von Volkmann R. Wer trägt den Taluskopf wirklich, und inwiefern ist der plantare Sehnenast des M. tibialis post. als Bandsystem aufzufassen? Anat Anz 1972;131: 425–32.

46. von Volkmann R. Ein Ligamentum "neglectum" pedis (Lig. calcaneonaviculare mediodorsale seu sustentaculonaviculare). Verh Anat Ges 1970;64:483–90.

47. von Volkmann R. Zur Anatomie und Mechanik des Lig. calcaneonaviculare plantare sensu strictori. Anat Anz 1973;134:460–70.

48. Hardy RH. Observations on the structure and properties of the calcaneonavicular ligament in man. J Anat 1951;85:135–9.

49. Mengiardi B, Pfirrmann CW, Vienne P, et al. Medial collateral ligament complex of the ankle: MR appearance in asymptomatic subjects. Radiology 2007;242: 817–24.

50. Hintermann B, Golanó P. The anatomy and function of the deltoid ligament. Tech Foot Ankle Surg 2014;13:62–72.

51. Cromeens BP, Kirchhoff CA, Patterson RM, et al. An attachment-based description of the medial collateral and spring ligament complexes. Foot Ankle Int 2015; 36:710–21.

52. Haynes JA, Gosselin M, Cusworth B, et al. The arterial anatomy of the deltoid ligament: a cadaveric study. Foot Ankle Int 2017;38:785–90.

53. Cahill DR. The anatomy and function of the contents of the human tarsal sinus and canal. Anat Rec 1965;153:1–18.

54. Laidlaw PP. The varieties of the os calcis. J Anat 1904;38:133–43.

55. Wood Jones F. The talocalcanean articulation. Lancet 1944;244(6312):241–2.

56. Wood Jones F. Structure and function as seen in the foot. London: Bailliére, Tindall & Cox; 1944.

57. Schwarzenbach B, Dora C, Lang A, et al. Blood vessels of the sinus tarsi and the sinus tarsi syndrome. Clin Anat 1997;10:173–82.

58. Retzius A. Bemerkungen über ein schlenderförmiges Band in dem Sinus tarsi des Menschen und mehrerer Thiere. Arch Anat Phys Wiss Med (Müller's Archiv) 1841;497–505.

59. Smith JW. The ligamentous structures in the canalis and sinus tarsi. J Anat 1958; 92:612–20.

60. Schmidt HM. Gestalt und Befestigung der Bandsysteme in Sinus und Canalis tarsi des Menschen. Acta Anat 1978;102:184–94.

61. Harper MC. The lateral ligamentous support of the subtalar joint. Foot Ankle 1991; 11:354–8.

62. Mabit C, Boncoeur-Martel MP, Chaudruc JB, et al. Anatomic and MRI study of the subtalar ligamentous support. Surg Radiol Anat 1997;19:111–7.

63. Stagni R, Leardini A, ÓConnor JJ, et al. Role of passive structures in the mobility and stability of the human subtalar joint: a literature review. Foot Ankle Int 2003; 24:402–9.

64. Jotoku T, Kinoshita M, Okuda R, et al. Anatomy of ligamentous structures in the tarsal sinus and canal. Foot Ankle Int 2006;27:533–8.

65. Li SY, Hou ZD, Zhang P, et al. Ligament structures in the tarsal sinus and canal. Foot Ankle Int 2013;34:1729–36.

66. Mulfinger GL, Trueta J. The blood supply of the talus. J Bone Joint Surg Br 1970; 52-B:160–7.

67. Champetier J. Innervation de Íarticulation tibio-tarsienne (Articulatio talocruralis). Acta Anat 1970;77:398–421.

68. Schmidt HM, Grünwald E. Untersuchungen an den Bandsystemen der talocruralen und intertarsalen Gelenke des Menschen. Gegenbaurs Morph Jahrb 1981; 127:792–831.

69. DiGiovanni CW, Langer PR, Nickisch F, et al. Proximity of the lateral talar process to the lateral stabilizing ligaments of the ankle and subtalar joint. Foot Ankle Int 2007;28:175–80.

70. Toldt K, Hochstetter F. Anatomischer Atlas. Erster Band. Berlin (Germany): Urban und Schwarzenberg; 1928.

71. Manter JT. Movements of the subtalar and transverse tarsal joint. J Anat 1941;80: 397–410.

72. Hicks J. The mechanics of the foot. I. The joints. J Anat 1953;87:345–57.

73. Zographos S, Chaminade B, Hobatho MC, et al. Experimental study of the subtalar joint axis preliminary investigation. Surg Radiol Anat 2000;22:271–6.

74. Seringe R, Wicart P. The talonavicular and subtalar joints: the "calcaneopedal unit" concept. Orthop Traumatol Surg Res 2013;99:S345–55.

75. Jastifer JR, Gustafson PA. The subtalar joint: biomechanics and functional repre-sentations in the literature. Foot (Edinb) 2014;24:203–9.
76. Maceira E, Monteagudo M. Subtalar anatomy and mechanics. Foot Ankle Clin N Am 2015;20:195–221.
77. Inman VT. The joints of the ankle. Baltimore (MD): Williams & Wilkins; 1976.
78. van Langelaan EJ. A kinematical analysis of the tarsal joints. An X-ray photogram-metric study. Acta Orthop Scand Suppl 1983;204:1–269.
79. MacConaill MA, Basmajian JV. Muscles and movements: a basis for human kine-siology. Baltimore (MD): Williams & Wilkins; 1969.

Subtalar Joint Biomechanics

From Normal to Pathologic

Adam Sangeorzan, MD[a],*, Bruce Sangeorzan, MD[b]

KEYWORDS

- Subtalar joint • Hindfoot mechanics • Valgus • Varus • Subtalar joint axis
- Peritalar joint • Flatfoot • Dynamic varus

KEY POINTS

- Subtalar joint function is driven by the complex shape of its articulations.
- Motion about the subtalar joint is triplanar and described using the terms *inversion/eversion*, *adduction/abduction*, and *plantarflexion/dorsiflexion*.
- Congenital or traumatic changes to the articulations of the subtalar joint can lead to alterations in function.
- The orientation of the subtalar joint axis may be a primary risk factor for development of pes planus.

ANATOMY OF THE PERITALAR JOINT

The subtalar joint consists of 2 articulations with separate synovial sheaths. The first is between the posterior facets of the talus and calcaneus (the posterior talocalcaneal joint [TCJ]). This is separated from the second sheath by the sinus tarsi, a sulcus formed between the posterior and medial facets of the talus and calcaneus, respectively, and filled with the strong talocalcaneal interosseous ligament. The second articulation is made up of the anterior and medial facets of the calcaneus and talus, talar head, the navicular bone, and the cartilaginous surface of the calcaneonavicular ligament (talocalcaneonavicular joint [TCNJ]). The TCNJ is described as the acetabulum pedis by some investigators because it (in conjunction with the fibrocartilage surface of the spring ligament and posterior tibial tendon) forms a socket (acetabulum) for the talar head about which the foot is able to move in 3 planes.[1-3] Although anatomically made up of 2 separate joint capsules, these articulations do not move independently

Disclosure: The authors have no disclosures of any commercial or financial interest in the subject matter or materials discussed in the article.
[a] Department of Orthopaedics and Sports Medicine, Harborview Medical Center, University of Washington, Box 359798, 325 9th Avenue, Seattle, WA 98104, USA; [b] Department of Orthopaedics and Sports Medicine, University of Washington, Seattle, WA, USA
* Corresponding author.
E-mail address: adams16@uw.edu

of one another.[1,4] Therefore, the distinction is artificial and orthopedic surgeons consider the TCJ and TCNJ 1 functional unit.[5]

Despite these anatomic distinctions, the peritalar joint is often described in the literature as the TCJ (all 3 facets of the talus and calcaneus as well as the fibrocartilage surface of the spring ligament) and the talonavicular joint (TNJ) (the articulation between the head of the talus and posterior surface of the navicular, which shares a synovial sheath with the anterior/middle facets of the calcaneus). The terms, *TNJ* and *TCJ*, are used for this discussion of biomechanics of the peritalar joint.[1] The TNJ and TCJ do not function independently of one another and, therefore, are referred to as the peritalar joint complex.

Also critical to discussing the biomechanics of the subtalar joint is establishing a common vernacular for describing motion about the joint. Unfortunately, much discrepancy exists in the literature. The human foot is unique, because it has evolved to be oriented perpendicular to the axis of the body to allow for bipedal locomotion. The subtalar joint axis is also obliquely oriented, resulting in complex triplanar motion. This means that terms used to describe motion at the subtalar joint are inexact and confusing. As such, the authors prefer to avoid terms like supination and pronation as applied to the subtalar joint. Throughout this article, frontal plane motion is described as inversion or eversion, transverse plane motion is described as adduction or abduction, and sagittal plane motion is described as plantar flexion or dorsiflexion (**Fig. 1**).

The unique triplanar motion of the subtalar joint is a direct result of the bony shape of the articular surfaces of the TCJ and the TNJ. These may be classified as male and female ovoid surfaces. The posterior facet of the calcaneus and the head of the talus are male ovoid surfaces whereas the middle and anterior calcaneal facets, the

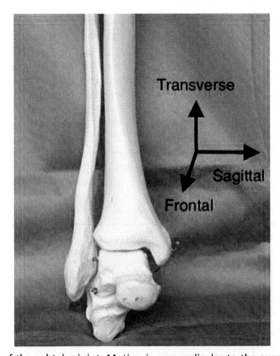

Fig. 1. The axes of the subtalar joint. Motion is perpendicular to the axes of the joint.

posterior facet of the talus, and the navicular are female ovoid surfaces.[1] This shape results in a complex twisting motion at the TCJ that can only occur as long as the anterior and medial facets can accommodate motion opposite to the motion at the posterior facet. The male ovoid surface moving on a female surface is that of a slide, roll, and spin where the direction of the slide is opposite of the direction of the roll. The female surface moving on a male surface has the same 3 planes of motion, but the role is in the same direction as the slide.[1,6] This slide and roll motion has been described as a screwlike. Manter[7] and Inman[8] both found on cadaveric specimens that, as the talus twists on the calcaneus, there is relative posterior displacement of the calcaneus on the talus. Inman found, however, that the displacement was not always linear and, therefore, does not describe linear increments, as would a screw. Therefore, most articles describe the subtalar joint as moving along a single axis, which is the convention used in this article.

Motion of the TNJ is closely coupled with and limited by the TCJ. The head of the talus articulates with the posterior surface of the navicular and is further supported by the plantar calcaneonavicular (spring) ligament, the deltoid ligament, bifurcate ligament, and the aforementioned anterior and middle facets of the calcaneus. These structures form the acetabulum pedis, cupping the talar head and leading to a near ball-and-socket joint configuration analogous to the hip. Because the TCJ and TNJ motion are coupled, this less constrained ball-and-socket joint is limited by the complex concave/convex relationship of the TCJ, as previously described,[3,5] and explains why TNJ motion is more limited than expected from a simpler ball-and-socket joint.

AXIS OF THE SUBTALAR/PERITALAR JOINT

The axis of rotation of the TCJ constrains the motion of the TNJ and leads to the triplanar motion of the subtalar/peritalar joint. The axis of both joints are described.

As discussed previously, the TCJ is most often considered a uniaxial joint with a single oblique axis of rotation that extends superiorly and medially from the talus. This axis was well described initially by Manter.[7] He studied 16 cadaveric feet and determined the TCJ axis was shifted on average 42° dorsally (29°–47°) in the sagittal plane and 16° (8°–24°) medially in the transverse plane compared with a line from the midpoint of the heel to the intersection between the first and second toes. Inman and Isman[8,9] studied a total of 102 feet in separate cadaveric studies and defined the sagittal plane as running from the midpoint of the heel to a bisection of the second and third toes. This study led to a TCJ axis of 42° ± 9° in the sagittal plane (20.5°–68.5°) and 23° ± 11° (4°–47°) in the transverse plane (**Fig. 2**).

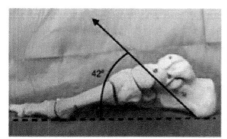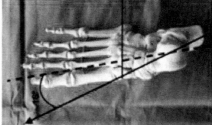

Fig. 2. The axis of the TCJ as described by Manter[7] in the sagittal (*left*) and transverse (*right*) planes. Dotted line was assigned as midline; solid line is the axis of the TCJ.

The axis of rotation of the subtalar joint points medially, anteriorly, and superiorly. This orientation allows motion primarily in the frontal (inversion/eversion) and transverse (adduction and abduction) plane. There is also a small amount of sagittal plane (flexion/extension) motion. This motion is primarily controlled by the more constrained TCJ, which guides motion of the TNJ.[3] Isman and Inman[9] found that the average range of motion of the TCJ was 18° ± 6°.

TCJ motion is triplanar: inversion, adduction, and plantar flexion occur together (down and in motion of acetabulum pedis) whereas eversion, abduction, and dorsiflexion occur together (up and out). Using these descriptive terms is the authors' preferred method of describing motion at the peritalar joint complex, because the terms, *pronation* and *supination*, can lead to ambiguity and there is disagreement on these terms in the literature. Technically pronation/supination would be the position the foot is in when the body is prone/supine. Another example is if the hindfoot is in valgus (pronated), the forefoot must be in supination to be flat to the floor. If the hindfoot is then corrected into varus (supination) and the forefoot maintains its relationship to the hindfoot, the medial forefoot would be off the ground and need to be "pronated" to be flat to the ground again. Therefore, the forefoot and hindfoot cannot be *pronated* or *supinated* at the same time and be in functional positions for stance or normal gait. For these reasons, we believe it is best to avoid the terminology of pronation/supination.

TNJ motion is also triplanar due to its close relationship to and constraint by the TCJ. Despite its shared synovial sheath with the anterior part of the TCJ, the TNJ is often considered part of the midtarsal joint in conjunction with the calcaneocuboid joint. Manter[7] determined that there 2 axes of rotation of the midtarsal joint. Compared with a line drawn from the heel to between the first and second toes, he described a longitudinal axis, inclined 15° superior from the floor and rotated 9° medially, and an oblique axis inclined 52° from the floor and 57° medially. Because the oblique axis is oriented more medially than the TCJ axis, there is more sagittal plane motion at the TNJ.[3]

MIDTARSAL JOINT LOCKING MECHANISM

Important to the discussion of subtalar joint biomechanics is the effect of hindfoot position on the rigidity of the foot. The foot becomes a rigid lever arm during forward propulsion and a mobile adaptor during weight acceptance. Elftman[10] postulated that the midtarsal joint (TNJ and calcaneocuboid joint) and the TCJ function in concert. When the hindfoot is in valgus/everted, the axis of the TCJ and midtarsal joint are in parallel, theoretically allowing for more motion in the midfoot and forefoot during weight acceptance. When the hindfoot/subtalar joint is inverted, the axes of the 2 joints converge, theoretically limiting motion of the forefoot and midfoot (**Fig. 3**). Blackwood and colleagues[11] performed a cadaveric study on 9 specimens in which they fixed the talus in place in relation to the tibia and tested forefoot and midfoot range of motion with the hindfoot in eversion, neutral, and inversion. They found significant increases in sagittal plane (dorsiflexion/plantarflexion) range of motion of the forefoot (first, second, and fifth metatarsals) when the calcaneus was everted compared with inverted. Surprisingly they found an insignificant increase in navicular sagittal plane motion as inversion of the hindfoot increased. There was no significant change in frontal or transverse plane motion of the forefoot or midfoot through the range of hindfoot position. They concluded that sagittal plane motion of the forefoot is increased with hindfoot eversion, allowing for a foot that can act as a rigid lever or an accommodative platform in different phases of gait, proving Elftman's proposal[10] that subtalar joint position critically influences the biomechanics of gait.

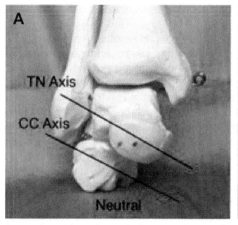
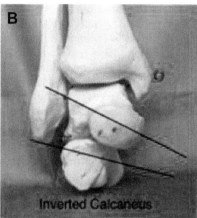

Fig. 3. The midtarsal joint locking mechanism from the frontal plane. In panel A, the TN and CC axes are in parallel with the calcaneus in neutral. In panel B, the calcaneus is inverted and the axes become convergent. Inversion of the calcaneus places the talar head above the CC join and limits motion of the midfoot.

JOINT KINETICS

Several investigators have studied the contact pressures in the TCJ, and to a lesser extent the TNJ. Wagner and colleagues[12] studied 13 cadaveric specimens using pressure sensitive film placed on the posterior and anteromedial facets of the calcaneus with increasing loads applied (300 N → 1400 N). This was done in positions of a neutral ankle, plantar, and dorsiflexion and in hindfoot positions of neutral, eversion, and inversion. There were several key findings:

1. As load increases, ratio of contact area to total joint area of the posterior facet increases.
2. As load increases, the ratio of high-pressure contact area to total contact area in the posterior facet increases.
3. When the hindfoot was positioned in inversion, there was significantly less contact area/total joint area in the posterior facet, but the same ratio of high-pressure contact area to total contact area.
4. The anterior/middle facet contact characteristics were not changed with foot position. Contact area/joint area and high-pressure contact area/contact area ratios increased with low load increases (350 N → 700 N) but not with subsequently higher loads.

These findings show that posterior facet contact pressures are affected by hindfoot position and suggest that inverted hindfoot position leads to higher pressures in the posterior facet.

Reeck and colleagues[13] expanded on this work, measuring TCJ pressures with Fuji film in heel strike, foot flat, and near toe-off on 14 cadaveric feet. They found that the posterior facet contact area increased from heel strike (477 mm^2) to toe-off (610 mm^2). There was an increase in mean joint contact pressure from 1.5 MPa at heel strike to 2.40 MPa at near toe-off as well as total force across the posterior facet from 685 N to 1492 N at near toe-off. There was no difference in contact area or pressure in the anteromedial facet but total force increased from 391 N at heel strike to 538 N at midstance. There is variation in the pressures found in the TCJ across studies, but there is agreement that pressures in the anteromedial and posterior facets range approximately from 0.93 MPa to 3.23 MPa.[12–15]

Rosenbaum and colleagues[15] also looked at the TNJ and found the loading force of the TNJ to be 119 N ±54 N over 68 mm² ±20 mm² for an average pressure of 1.75 MPa. Reeck and colleagues[13] found that the contact area of the TNJ did not change from heel strike to midstance but increased from 382 mm² to 441 mm² at near toe-off. There was no change in contact pressures in the TNJ for different phases of gait but there was an increase in contact force from midstance to near toe-off. They found contact pressures of approximately 2 MPa.

CONTACT CHARACTERISTICS OF THE SUBTALAR JOINT AFTER TRAUMA

As outlined previously, subtalar joint function is intimately related to the osteology of the articular surfaces. It stands to reasons that alteration in the shape of the surfaces after fracture would alter biomechanics. Sangeorzan and colleagues[16] simulated talar neck misalignment in 7 cadaveric specimens and measured contact characteristics of the posterior and anteromedial calcaneal facets using pressure sensitive film. One of the films measured pressures greater than 0.5 MPa to detect total contact area. The other film was only able to detect pressures greater than 6 MPa and determined high-pressure zone areas. They tested pressures prior to talar neck osteotomy, postosteotomy with anatomic reduction, and 2 mm of displacement medially, laterally and with varus angulation and dorsal displacement respectively. They found the following:

1. There were no significant changes in the posterior facet in terms of contact area (mean normal = 536 mm²) or mean high-pressure zone area (mean normal = 66 mm²) for any of the talar neck positions tested.
2. The contact print on the posterior facet changed from a more distributed to more localized total contact area with nonanatomic reduction of the neck. Meaning the same force was distributed in a smaller area with talar neck displacement.
3. There were no significant changes in contact area of the anteromedial facet. Mean total contact area was similar in normal and nondisplaced osteotomies (131 mm² and 135 mm²), however, but decreased to a mean of 81 mm² and 56 mm² with lateral and dorsal displacement.
4. There were no significant differences in high-pressure zone areas between normal and nondisplaced osteotomies in the anteromedial facets. All of the displaced fractures, however, demonstrated significant unloading of the anteromedial facets.

The investigators concluded that 2-mm changes in talar neck alignment lead to off-loading of the anteromedial facet without transfer of more pressure to the posterior facet. This suggests that talar neck malalignment leads to this additional load being transmitted through an alternate path, such as the TNJ, or an extra-articular pathway, such as impingement in the sinus tarsi. This could lead to pain and degenerative arthrosis and supports the guideline of fixing fractures with 2 mm of displacement.

Using similar techniques, Sangeorzan and colleagues[17] examined 9 cadaveric specimens in which a calcaneus fracture through the posterior facet was simulated. They tested in positions of anatomic reduction and displacements of 2 mm, 5 mm, and 10 mm. The contact area was significantly decreased for 2-mm, 5-mm, and 10-mm displacements (mean of 349.4 mm² initially compared with 280 mm² with 2 mm of displacement). The high-pressure area in the posterior facet was only significantly increased with displacement of 5 mm and 10 mm (3.6 mm² in normal joint vs 12.9 mm² in displacement of 5 mm). The anatomically reduced simulated fractures showed no significant changes in total contact area or high-pressure area compared with the normal posterior facet. There were no significant changes observed in the anteromedial facets at any displacement. The investigators concluded that fixing fractures displaced 2 mm was supported by their findings and that the increased high-pressure contact area seen with displacement could lead to pain and arthrosis.

HINDFOOT VALGUS

Most literature on symptomatic adult flatfoot is focused on the contribution of soft tissue support to the medial column, such as the posterior tibial tendon, the talonavicular capsule, the spring ligament, and the contribution of Achilles overpull. These are important contributors but do not define the underlying cause. And although the axis of rotation of the subtalar joint has been defined over the years, only recently with technological improvements allowing 3-D mapping of bone surfaces[18,19] has the literature supported variations in the shape of the bone by foot type and imputed a difference in axis in patients with hindfoot valgus. Years ago, Dyal and colleagues noted that the nonsymptomatic foot in patients treated for symptomatic flat foot often had bony landmarks similar to those of the symptomatic foot although without symptoms.[20] Little was made of that recognition until computer technology advanced to be able to recreate volume maps of individual bones of individual people from DICOM (Digital Imaging and Communications in Medicine) data of CT images.

Ananthakrisnan and colleagues[21] first demonstrated actual subluxation of the subtalar joint in patients with symptomatic flatfoot compared with normal controls using weight-bearing CT scan and volume maps of the joint services. By comparing the position of the talar and calcaneal surfaces in painful flat feet to normal control patients, they showed posterior and lateral subluxation of the posterior facet of the calcaneus relative to that of the talus. The posterior facet of the calcaneus moved more than the middle facet. Although the middle facet moved less, it demonstrated gapping between the bones consistent with the tilt of the calcaneus around the sinus tarsi.

Both intrinsic (bone morphology) and extrinsic (bone position) differences exist in groups of feet described as cavus and planus.[19] Although bone morphology was different in different foot types, concrete clinical correlation was not called out. Apostle and colleagues[22] compared the shape and orientation of the posterior facet of the subtalar joint using weight-bearing CT scans. They compared 22 feet in 20 patients undergoing reconstruction for painful flatfoot to 20 feet in a control group. They measured the angle between the superior talar dome and posterior facet of the talus on coronal CT scan from anterior to posterior in both groups. They excluded patients with severe subtalar arthritis and patients with stage 4 flatfoot because of tilt of the talus in the ankle mortise confounding their findings. They found that the axis of the symptomatic flatfoot started in valgus and became more valgus from anterior to posterior. The normal feet started in varus anteriorly and progressed to much more mild valgus. There was a significant difference at the mean, maximum, and minimum valgus values, showing the symptomatic flat feet had a more valgus subtalar axis in all areas (flat feet showed an average minimum of 3.6° of valgus and maximum of 34° of valgus whereas normal controls mean minimum value was 5.8° of varus to a mean maximum of 18° degrees of valgus). The investigators hypothesized that a valgus subtalar axis is a congenital risk factor and perhaps the primary cause for development of adult acquired flatfoot. They also suggested a new treatment option for treating adult flatfoot would be an opening wedge subarticular osteotomy of the talus to improve joint orientation and address the true cause of deformity. Both Apostle and colleagues[22] and Probasco and colleagues[23] measured this coronal plane subtalar joint alignment and hypothesized that the excessive valgus angulation of the subtalar joint led to a force vector that caused stress over time to the medial soft tissue structures, leading to their failure and progression of deformity (**Fig. 4**).

In its most advanced stage, the translation of the posterior facet can lead to atraumatic subtalar dislocation in which the calcaneus translates until it is primarily under the fibula rather than the talus and causes subfibular impingement (**Fig. 5**). Ramadorai and colleagues[24] presented their data on 23 patients. They defined atraumatic dislocation based on CT criteria (3 consecutive sagittal CT cuts of the calcaneus without the talus, 3 consecutive sagittal cuts of the talus without the calcaneus, and presence of a calcaneofibular articulation).

Based on these data the authors believe that a valgus subtalar joint axis leads to altered force vectors about the foot and ankle that place unusually high stresses on the medial soft tissues of the ankle, hypothesizing that this altered axis is the primary cause of adult acquired flatfoot.

CAVUS, VARUS, AND DYNAMIC VARUS

The subtalar joint plays an important role in hindfoot varus, cavus foot, and dynamic varus. The terms, *cavus foot* and *pes cavus*, are used to describe a less flexible foot with a high arch, a varus hindfoot, and compensatory changes in the forefoot. Although a flexible forefoot driven cavus is marked by hyperplantar flexion of the first ray, a rigid cavus is characterized by derotation of the TCJ combined with a joint shape that creates a more inward axis.

When the AP talocalcaneal angle is narrow, the talar head is superior to the anterior process of the calcaneus, which imposes a similar position on Chopart joint with the navicular resting on the cuboid. That limits motion of the midfoot particularly in the sagittal plane (**Fig. 6**).[25]

DYNAMIC VARUS

The opposite of the valgus subtalar axis, described previously, is a varus tilted axis. Dynamic varus is not the same as subtle cavus. Dynamic varus describes a clinical situation in which the hindfoot appears neutral when standing comfortably but does not

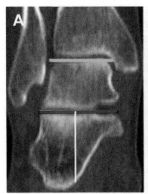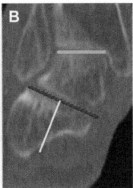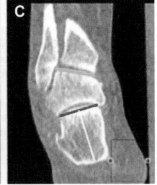

Fig. 4. Normal to pathologic: the coronal alignment of the subtalar joint drives hindfoot position. These are simulated weight bearing CT scans of patients with a neutral hindfoot (*A*), valgus hindfoot (*B*), and varus hindfoot (*C*), showing neutral, valgus and varus subtalar joint axes respectively. The white line represents a plumb line perpendicular to the subtalar joint.

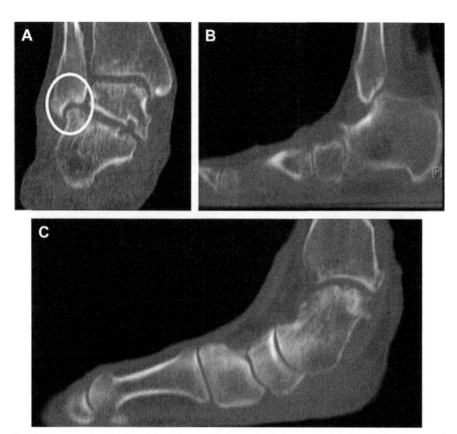

Fig. 5. Atraumatic subtalar dislocation: end stage of adult acquired flat foot showing a cal-caneofibular articulation (*A, white circle*) and a sagittal cut of the calcaneus without the talus (*B*) and talus without the calcaneus (*C*).

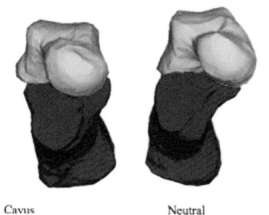

Cavus   Neutral

Fig. 6. 3-D model showing (*left*) a varus hindfoot with a tight talocalcaneal axis. The talar head is above the anterior process of the calcaneus and limits motion of the midfoot, anal-ogous to the midtarsal joint locking mechanism (discussed previously). (*Right*) A neutral hindfoot with a more divergent talocalcaneal axis.

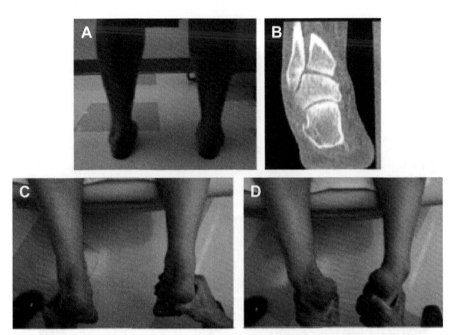

Fig. 7. Clinical example of a patient with dynamic varus. The patient has neutral alignment when standing (*A*). Image (*B*) represents a weight-bearing CT scan with a varus tilt to the subtalar joint axis. The standing alignment is actually the maximum valgus these patients can achieve (*C*) and all functional motion is in inversion from that point (*D*).

evert beyond neutral. The standing neutral position represents the fully everted position of the joint. The hindfoot does not evert from that position. It should be considered in patients with recurrent sprains and those who have failed lateral ligament reconstruction but do not appear to have varus. Patients with dynamic varus do not have a high arch, a plantar flexed first ray, or the appearance of varus while standing. In this subgroup the hindfoot has a varus axis but at its maximum valgus, which is the standing position, they are neutral. But on examination, they do not evert beyond neutral and invert 30° or greater (**Fig. 7**).

SUMMARY

In conclusion, subtalar joint biomechanics are primarily driven by the shape of the articulations between the talus, calcaneus, and navicular bone, with contributions from the surrounding soft tissues. The motions about the TCJ and TNJ are triplanar and can be described by the terms inversion/eversion, adduction/abduction, and plantarflexion/dorsiflexion. Joint contact forces change during different stages of gait and are affected by hindfoot alignment and traumatic alterations to their normal anatomy. The authors believe that the subtalar joint axis is a contributing, and perhaps primary, risk factor for progression to adult acquired flat foot and that the axis also contributes to the clinical picture of a cavus foot and a special subset of patients with dynamic varus.

REFERENCES

1. Sarraffian SK. Biomechanics of the subtalar joint complex. Clin Orthop Relat Res 1993;(290):17–26.

2. Mosca V. Principles of management of pediatric foot and ankle deformities and malformations. Wolters Kluwer; 2014.
3. Ledoux WR, Sangeorzan BJ. Clinical biomechanics of the peritalar joint. Foot Ankle Clin 2004;9(4):663–83.
4. Lapidus PW. Subtalar joint, its anatomy and mechanics. Bull Hosp Jt Dis 1955;16: 179–95.
5. Rockar PA. The subtalar joint: anatomy and joint motion. J Orthop Sports Phys Ther 1995;21(6):361–72.
6. MacConaill MA, Basmajian J. Muscles and movements: a basis for human kinesiology. Baltimore (MD): Williams & Wilkins; 1969. p. 23.
7. Manter JT. Movements of the subtalar and transverse tarsal joints. Anat Rec 1941; 80(4):397–410.
8. Inman VT. The joints of the ankle. Baltimore (MD): Williams and Wilkins; 1976.
9. Isman RE, Inman VT. Anthropometric studies of the human foot and ankle. San Francisco (CA): Biomechanics laboratory, University of California; 1968. San Francisco and Berkely.
10. Elftman H. The transverse tarsal joint and its control. Clin Orthop 1960;14:41–5.
11. Blackwood B, Yuen T, Sangeorzan B, et al. The midtarsal joint locking mechanism. Foot Ankle Int 2005;26:1074–80.
12. Wagner U, Sangeorzan B, Harrington R, et al. Contact characteristics of the subtalar joint: load distribution between the anterior and posterior facets. J Orthop Res 1992;10:535–43.
13. Reeck J, Felten N, McCormack AP, et al. Support of the talus: a biomechanical investigation of the contributions of the talonavicular and talocalcaneal joints, and the superomedial calcaneonavicular ligament. Foot Ankle Int 1998;19(10): 674–82.
14. Wang CL, Cheng CK, Chen CW, et al. Contact areas and pressure distributions in the subtalar join. J Biomech 1995;28(3):269–79.
15. Rosenbaum D, Bertsch C, Claes LE. NOVEL award 1996: 2nd prize tenodeses do not fully restore ankle joint loading characteristics: a biomechanical in vitro investigation in the hind foot. Clin Biomech 1997;12(3):202–9.
16. Sangeorzan B, Wagner U, Harrington R, et al. Contact characteristics of the subtalar joint: the effect of talar neck misalignment. J Orthop Res 1992;10:544–51.
17. Sangeorzan B, Ananthakrishnan D, Tencer A. Contact characteristics of the subtalar joint after a simulated calcaneus fracture. J Orthop Trauma 1995;9(3):251–8.
18. Ledoux WR, Rohr ES, Ching RP, et al. Effect of foot shape on the three dimensional position of foot bones. J Orthop Res 2006;24:2176–86.
19. Louie PK, Sangeorzan BJ, Fassbind MJ, et al. Talonavicular joint coverage and bone morphology between different foot types. J Orthop Res 2014;32(7):958–66.
20. Dyal CM, Feder J, Deland JT, et al. Pes planus in patients with posterior tibial tendon insufficiency: asymptomatic versus symptomatic foot. Foot Ankle Int 1997;18(2):85–8.
21. Ananthakrisnan D, Ching R, Hansen ST Jr, et al. Subluxation of the talocalcaneal joints in adults who have symptomatic flatfoot. J Bone Joint Surg Am 1999;81(8): 1147–54.
22. Apostle K, Coleman N, Sangeorzan BJ. Subtalar joint axis in patients with symptomatic peritalar subluxation compared to normal controls. Foot Ankle Int 2014; 35(11):1153–8.
23. Probasco W, Haleem A, Yu J, et al. Assessment of coronal plane subtalar joint alignment in peritalar subluxation via weight-bearing multiplanar imaging. Foot Ankle Int 2015;36(3):302–9.

24. Ramadorai U, Williams J, Sangeorzan BJ. Treatment of atraumatic subtalar dislocations in adult acquired flatfoot deformity. AOFAS Annual Meeting. Ontario, July 20–23, 2016.
25. Aminian A, Sangeorzan BJ. The anatomy of cavus foot deformity. Foot Ankle Clin 2008;13(2):191–8.

Traumatic Injury to the Subtalar Joint

Stefan Rammelt, MD, PhD[a],*, Jan Bartoníček, MD, DSc[b], Kyeong-Hyeon Park, MD[c]

KEYWORDS

- Subtalar dislocation • Talar fracture • Calcaneal fracture • Sustentacular fracture
- Talar process fracture • Cartilage • Arthritis

KEY POINTS

- Traumatic injury to the subtalar joint disrupts normal hindfoot motion and potentially leads to restricted global foot function.
- The subtalar joint is injured during subtalar dislocations, talar and calcaneal fractures, and fracture-dislocations.
- Anatomic reconstruction of joint congruity is essential for functional rehabilitation after subtalar joint injury.
- Failure to anatomically reduce the subtalar joint potentially leads to chronic instability, subtalar arthritis, and posttraumatic hindfoot deformity.

INTRODUCTION

The subtalar joint plays a central role in load transmission and movement at the hindfoot, especially when adapting the foot to uneven ground surfaces. Traumatic injury to the subtalar joint disrupts normal hindfoot motion and may significantly restrict global foot function.[1]

The anatomy of the subtalar joint is complex. The posterior part (talocalcaneal joint) is composed of the posterior talar and calcaneal facets. The anterior part (talocalcaneonavicular joint) consists of the anterior and middle facets of the calcaneus, the posterior concave facet of the navicular bone, the spring ligament between the navicular bone, and the calcaneus, as well and the corresponding joint facets of the talus. Both

Disclosure Statement: The authors do not have any relationship with a commercial company that has a direct financial interest in subject matter or materials discussed in article or with a company making a competing product.

[a] Foot & Ankle Section, University Center for Orthopaedics and Traumatology, University Hospital Carl Gustav Carus at the TU Dresden, Fetscherstrasse 74, Dresden 01307, Germany; [b] Department of Orthopaedics, First Faculty of Medicine, Charles University, Central Military Hospital Prague, U Vojenské nemocnice 1200, Prague 6 169 02, Czech Republic; [c] Department of Orthopedic Surgery, Kyungpook National University Hospital, 130 Dongdeok-ro, Jung-gu, Daegu 41944, Korea
* Corresponding author.
E-mail address: strammelt@hotmail.com

structures are divided by the sinus and canalis tarsi (tarsal canal), which contains the talocalcaneal interosseous ligament complex. The subtalar joint is stabilized by its natural bony structure and reinforced by numerous ligaments within the sinus tarsi, the tarsal canal, the posterior subtalar joint, and the talonavicular joint. The osseous structure of the joint itself is the most important inherent stabilizer of the joint. Because of its oblique axis, motion within the subtalar joint is 3-dimensional and properly summarized as inversion (lifting the inner margin of the foot = supination, internal rotation, and plantarflexion) and eversion (lifting the outer margin of the foot = pronation, external rotation, and dorsiflexion) of the midfoot and forefoot (the subtalar plate) with respect to the hindfoot.[2,3]

The subtalar joint acts in conjunction with the talonavicular and calcaneocuboid joints while forming the triple joint complex. Normal function of the subtalar joint is critical for the ability of the foot to accommodate uneven or irregular surfaces. In addition, it bears an integral proprioceptive function of the foot and ankle.[3,4]

Intraarticular fractures of the talus or calcaneus lead to cartilaginous defects and displacement of the articular surface. Displaced extraarticular fractures of the talus and calcaneus result in axial deviation and, therefore, eccentric loading of the subtalar joint. Subtalar and talonavicular dislocations result from rotational and shearing forces, and are frequently accompanied by peripheral fractures of the talus and calcaneus.[5] Malalignment and instability of the subtalar joint alter the load distribution within the joint complex and potentially lead to subtalar arthrosis with pain and impaired function.[6] In contrast, posttraumatic arthrosis with dysfunction of the subtalar joint may be the result of direct injury to the cartilage by grinding or shearing forces during dislocations, or secondary chondrocyte apoptosis resulting from compressive forces or avascular necrosis (AVN) in severe fractures.[1,7] Relevant chondral injuries leading to degenerative changes are more likely to occur after dislocations accompanied by peripheral fractures than after pure dislocations of the subtalar joint.[8] In the following, the 3 main traumatic injuries to the subtalar joint will be discussed with respect to the pathomechanism, evaluation and management:

- Subtalar dislocations with peripheral talar and calcaneal fractures;
- Central talar fractures with subtalar joint involvement; and
- Calcaneal fractures with subtalar joint involvement.

All of these injuries carry an intrinsic risk of posttraumatic arthritis for the abovementioned reasons. However, not all patients with radiographic evidence of arthritis become symptomatic and require subsequent fusion (**Table 1**).

Overall, there is a wide variety in the numbers for posttraumatic arthritis. The lowest rates of both arthritis and secondary fusion are seen after purely ligamentous subtalar dislocations.[5,8] Posttraumatic arthritis increases over time and reaches 100% with

Table 1
Rates of posttraumatic arthritis and secondary fusions after traumatic injury to the subtalar joint

Type of Injury	Subtalar Arthritis (%)	Subtalar Fusion (%)	References
Subtalar dislocations	39–89	0–26	5,8,12,14,16,18,27,36,109,110
Talar neck and body fractures	16–100	3–18	3,31,51–56,111–115
Intraarticular calcaneal fractures	5–100	0–32	3,59,67,73,74,76,94,101,102,116

longer follow-up after both talar and calcaneal fractures. In the treatment of intraartic-ular calcaneal fractures, the need for secondary subtalar fusion is increased 7-fold when considering nonoperative treatment.[3]

Combined talar and calcaneal fractures: Combined talar and calcaneal fractures are the most severe injuries to the subtalar joint. They are rare and display a very var-iable pattern of injury.[9,10] In particular, high rates of primary and secondary subtalar fusions are reported after closed injuries and up to 54% below-the-knee amputa-tions after combined open talar and calcaneal fractures, which constitute complex foot trauma.[9,11]

SUBTALAR DISLOCATIONS WITH PERIPHERAL TALAR AND CALCANEAL FRACTURES
Etiology

A subtalar dislocation is defined as a simultaneous dislocation of the subtalar (talocal-caneal) and talonavicular joints. Subtalar dislocations represent about 1% or 2% of all dislocations and 15% of all peritalar injuries.[12,13] In about 50% to 80% of cases, they are caused by high-energy injuries including motor vehicle accidents and falls from heights.[14–16] However, a considerable number of subtalar dislocations result from rather insignificant, low-energy injuries like severe hindfoot sprains or during sports.[17] About 75% of all reported cases are medial subtalar dislocations.[12,18,19] They are caused by forced inversion of the plantarflexed foot with the sustentaculum tali serving as a lever for the talar neck. In contrast, lateral subtalar dislocations make up 17% to 26% of the reported cases in larger series and are produced by forced eversion with the foot in dorsiflexion.[12,18,19] Anterior and posterior dislocations are rare, averaging 1% and 2% of all subtalar dislocations.[12,18] Anterior subtalar dislocations are most likely produced by anterior traction of the foot with the lower leg being fixed, whereas posterior subtalar dislocations are caused by heavy plantarflexion of the foot.[20,21] A total talar dislocation (luxatio tali totalis) is the extreme form of peritalar ligamentous injuries. In those injuries, the talus is disrupted from all its joints and dislocates completely. Leitner[19] regarded subtalar dislocations as a first stage to total talar dis-locations, which would result from continuing inversion stress on the ankle joint in medial or lateral subtalar dislocations. Indeed, subluxation at the ankle can be seen in severe forms of subtalar dislocations.[5]

Subtalar dislocations have to be distinguished from dislocations at the midtar-sal (Chopart) joint.[22] The talonavicular joint as part of the coxa pedis (the talocal-caneonavicular joint including the anterior chamber of the subtalar joint) is affected under both conditions. The main mechanism of injury at the midtarsal joint is an abduction or adduction dislocation force in conjunction with longitudi-nal compression.[23]

Subtalar dislocations are frequently associated with bony injuries. Most likely, these are peripheral fractures of the talus and calcaneus including fractures of the talar head, the lateral or posterior process of the talus, and the sustentaculum tali of the calcaneus. They may rapidly progress into painful posttraumatic arthritis of the subtalar joint.[5,8,24,25]

Diagnosis and Management

Medial dislocations display a medially displaced heel, inversion, and plantarflexion of the foot. Lateral dislocations typically result from a high-energy trauma and are more frequently associated with open injuries.[14] The heel is displaced laterally and the foot is in inversion and abduction. The deformity is less pronounced in posterior or anterior dislocations because there is less axial malalignment, but the susceptible skin over the foot may be put under tension.[20,21] The diagnosis can be confirmed using anteroposterior and lateral radiographs. Associated fractures of the lateral or posterior process of the talus and the sustentaculum tali of the calcaneus may be difficult to detect clinically because the pain is regularly projected over the ligaments and these fractures are regularly missed on plain radiographs. Dislocations and fracture-dislocations at the talonavicular joint are frequently associated with talar head or navicular fractures.[22] The clinical and pathognomonic sign is a plantar ecchymosis.

Early reduction of subtalar dislocations

Early reduction of subtalar dislocations is essential to avoid further damage to the soft tissues and neurovascular compromise (**Fig. 1**). If performed promptly, the majority of acute subtalar dislocations can be reduced in a closed manner under sedation, although a delayed reduction may require general anesthesia and proper muscle relaxation. In approximately 10% of medial subtalar dislocations, closed reduction is impossible. Open reduction via an anterolateral or oblique (Ollier's) lateral approach directly over the palpable talar head is indicated in irreducible injuries.[5] The tibialis posterior or the flexor digitorum longus tendon is slung around the talar head and prevents closed reduction in up to 40% of reported cases. In these instances, open reduction via an anterolateral (alternatively Ollier's) approach becomes necessary. After reduction, the lateral talar process should be checked for an associated fracture or interposed bony or cartilaginous avulsion. Anterior and posterior subtalar dislocations are reduced with axial traction to the affected foot while holding the knee flexed. After successful reduction, the foot is immobilized in a cast for 6 weeks. Temporary K-wire transfixation of the subtalar joint for 6 weeks is reserved for rare cases of marked

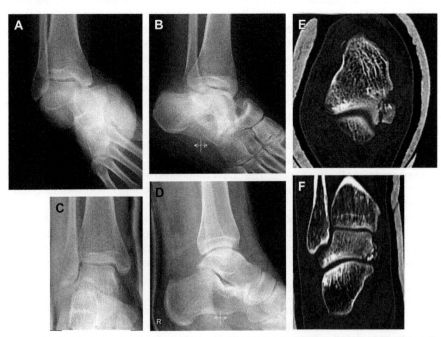

Fig. 1. (*A, B*) Medial subtalar dislocation. (*C, D*) Anteroposterior and lateral radiographs after closed reduction and external fixation. (*E, F*) Postreduction computed tomography scanning reveals a congruent subtalar joint and a minimally displaced, extraarticular posteromedial process fracture of the talus that is treated nonoperatively.

instability after initial reduction.[3] Because in more than 50% of cases subtalar dislocations are associated with talar process fractures and other peritalar injuries, computed
tomography (CT) scanning is necessary after successful closed reduction to detect or
rule out any other injuries to the talus and calcaneus (see **Fig. 1**; **Fig. 2**).[5,15,24]

Displaced lateral or posterior talar process fractures

Displaced lateral or posterior talar process fractures are either fixed anatomically or
removed if not amenable to internal fixation.[3] The lateral process is best accessed
via an oblique lateral (Ollier's) approach, whereas the posterior process is best visualized through a posterolateral or posteromedial approach. The subtalar and ankle joints
are cleared from debris and the size, location, and integrity of the fragments are
assessed. The fragments are fixed anatomically by means of minifragment screws
(2.0–2.7 mm; see **Fig. 2**). Alternatively, K-wires or resorbable pins may be used. Nonunions of the lateral or posterior process are best treated by resection of the fragments.[6]

Malalignment of the lateral and posterior process almost invariably results in
dysfunction of the subtalar joint and may rapidly progress to subtalar arthritis.[6,26,27]
In malunited posterior process fractures, and depending on the size and displacement
of the fragment, both the ankle and subtalar joints may be affected.[28] Comminuted

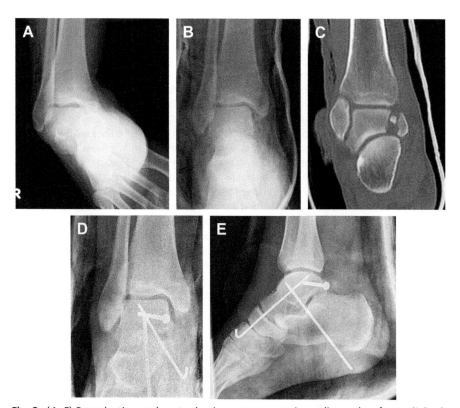

Fig. 2. (*A, B*) Prereduction and postreduction anteroposterior radiographs of a medial subtalar dislocation. (*C*) Postreduction computed tomography scanning reveals a displaced posterior process fracture of the talus with an intercalary fragment. (*D, E*) The posterior process
fracture is fixed with a screw via a posteromedial approach. Additional temporary transfixation of the subtalar joint is carried out because of gross postreduction instability.

fractures, especially those with a high degree of cartilage damage, and fragments not amenable to anatomic reduction, have to be excised to avoid joint irritation and progressive arthritis. Biomechanical studies have suggested that up to 10 mm of the lateral process of the talus may be resected without the risk of subtalar instability.[29] A loose os trigonum or bipartite talus may mimic a fracture nonunion of the posterior process.[30] Symptomatic ossicles are resected.[28,30]

Talar head fractures

Talar head fractures are accessed through a curved anteromedial incision extending from the medial malleolus to the navicular tuberosity. The superficial fascia is opened and the posterior tibial tendon pulled plantarly. By so doing, the medial plantar aspect of the talocalcaneonavicular joint is exposed. If the fracture extends far laterally, an additional anterolateral approach distally and medially to the sinus tarsi is performed to gain access to the lateral aspect of the talonavicular joint.[22]

Fractures of the talar head are fixed according to the individual fracture pattern with resorbable pins, K-wires, small fragment screws, or small curved 2.7-mm interlocking plates bridging the talar head to the talar neck and body.[31] If, for stability reasons, screws are introduced near or through the joint surface, the heads have to be countersunk. Alternatively, headless screws may be used. Interfragmentary compression is not desirable to avoid shortening of the talar head.[22]

Fractures of the sustentaculum tali

Fractures of the sustentaculum tali of the calcaneus are accessed via a small medial approach that lies directly above the palpable sustentaculum approximately 2 cm below and 1 cm in front of the medial malleolus and behind the navicular tuberosity.[25] Compared with the McReynolds medial approach to the calcaneus, this approach is located superiorly and reduces the risk of damage to the tibial neurovascular bundle.[3] The posterior tibial tendon is retracted dorsally and the floor of the tendon sheath is detached carefully from the periosteum. The medial aspect of the subtalar joint can now be inspected directly and any fractures of the sustentaculum tali and/or the medial facet of the talocalcaneonavicular joint are reduced under direct vision.[3] Preparation should not extend behind the sustentaculum, so as not to injure the deltoid branches of the posterior tibial artery that carry a substantial portion of the blood supply to the talar body.[32] Fixation of the sustentaculum tali is typically carried out with screws.[25] With extension of the fracture along the medial calcaneal wall, a small plate might be considered for fixation.[33]

Up to 40% of all subtalar dislocations are open injuries with lateral dislocations being more frequently affected.[8,14,34] These injuries require debridement of heavily contaminated and necrotic tissue, copious lavage, open reduction and fixation of associated fractures via the existing wound or an extension of the latter, and preferably tibiometatarsal external fixation for soft tissue consolidation.[5]

Results and Complications

Skin necrosis can potentially be avoided when acting quickly to reduce the dislocation. AVN of the talus has been noted after both medial and lateral subtalar dislocations. The reported rates range between 0% and 10% in closed dislocations and up to 50% for open dislocations.[12,14] Recent studies revealed that the rates could be reduced to 10% with aggressive management with early reduction and stable fixation.[35] Neurovascular deficits may result from direct damage to the peripheral nerves through traction or open wounds, or incarceration of the deep posterior neurovascular bundle, especially in lateral dislocations. Tendon lacerations can occur after interposition, above all the posterior tibial tendon, in lateral dislocations, potentially leading to posttraumatic tendinitis and dysfunction. Chronic ligamentous instability and recurrent subluxation after subtalar dislocations is rare and may be due to early motion and immobilization of less than 4 weeks' duration.[12] The reported rates of posttraumatic arthritis of the subtalar joint vary considerably between 39% and 89%, with the lowest rates being observed after purely ligamentous injuries.[3,5,36] Fewer than one-third of these patients become symptomatic and warrant secondary subtalar fusion.[8,37]

Prognosis after subtalar dislocation depends on the type of injury. Although purely ligamentous dislocations carry a good to excellent prognosis with early reduction,[36] less favorable results are seen with associated osseous and cartilaginous injuries.[5,8,12] Other negative prognostic factors include open subtalar dislocations and total talar dislocations.[14] However, even for the latter, early replantation may result in favorable results.[38] With respect to the trauma mechanism, excellent functional results are reported in up to 100% after low-energy injuries, although these numbers decrease to 15% with high-energy injuries.[14,17]

CENTRAL TALAR FRACTURES WITH SUBTALAR JOINT INVOLVEMENT
Etiology

Fractures of the talar body and neck are grouped as central fractures, in contrast with peripheral fractures of the talar head, the lateral and posterior process.[39,40] Central talar fractures are severe injuries because considerable forces are needed to break the strong cortical shell of the talus. They typically occur after high-energy trauma and are frequently associated with multiple injuries or polytrauma, which make treatment even more challenging. About two-thirds of the talar surface is covered with articular cartilage. Consequently, the majority of talar fractures are intraarticular. This pathomechanism explains the high risk of osteoarthritis after talar fractures. Many authors have demonstrated a relation between posttraumatic hindfoot malalignment or osteonecrosis and osteoarthritis.[41–43] Consequently, malunions and nonunions of the talus almost invariably result in posttraumatic arthritis and severe dysfunction of the foot.[6] Anatomic reduction and restoration of the anatomic axes are important to regain normal or near-normal function of the foot. However, arthritis of the subtalar joint can occur in the absence of osteonecrosis or joint incongruity. The cartilage may be damaged from the initial injury, prolonged immobilization, or underlying bone necrosis.[44]

Diagnosis and Management

A clinical diagnosis of central talar fractures usually is straightforward with a history of high-energy trauma, accompanying soft tissue damage, the inability to bear weight, joint dysfunction, and in cases of fracture-dislocation severe deformity with tethering of the skin through displaced fragments. The diagnosis is verified using plain radiographs. However, in suspected or confirmed talar fractures, a CT scan provides 3-dimensional data to understand the pattern of injury and helps to elaborate a treatment plan. In cases of acute fracture-dislocations, the CT scan is performed after gross reduction of the main fragments.

The subtalar joint is directly involved in fractures of the talar body. The distinction between talar neck and body fractures is made with sagittal CT scans. By definition, talar neck fractures run through the sinus tarsi, whereas talar body fractures extend into the lateral talar process and thus into the subtalar jont.[45] Undisplaced fractures of the talar neck and body, as confirmed by CT scan, can be treated nonoperatively. The hindfoot is held in a neutrally positioned cast. Alternatively, stable internal fixation with minimal incision allows for functional aftertreatment and reduces the risk of redislocation or nonunion.[32,40,46]

Unless there are no contraindications for surgery, all displaced talar neck and body fractures should be slated for open anatomic reduction and stable internal fixation. Fracture-dislocations have to be treated as emergencies. Gross dislocations are reduced immediately to prevent severe damage to the soft tissues and blood supply to the talar body (**Fig. 3**). Closed or percutaneous reduction under sufficient analgesia and relaxation may be attempted. Open fractures and fracture-dislocations are treated as emergencies according to the general treatment principles for open injuries with debridement, copious lavage, and tibiometatarsal transfixation after gross reduction and provisional internal fixation.

Fractures of the talar neck and body
Fractures of the talar neck and body are generally accessed via bilateral approaches to ensure anatomic reduction of the ankle and subtalar joints and to avoid axial malalignment or rotation.[32,40] The lateral incision allows control of reduction of the subtalar joint and is performed either as a straight or slightly curved incision starting from the tip of the fibula and running toward the sinus tarsi and lateral aspect of the talar neck. Alternatively, an oblique incision is carried out over the sinus tarsi in front of the lateral malleolus along the skin crests (Ollier's approach). In the superior part of the incision, the course of the lateral branch of the superficial peroneal nerve has to be preserved. In the inferior part of the incision, the peroneal tendons are mobilized and held away plantarly within their common tendon sheet with a soft strap. The inferior extensor retinaculum is dissected and the extensor digitorum brevis muscle is dissected from the anterior calcaneal process and held away bluntly. To gain insight into the subtalar joint, the lateral talocalcaneal ligament is dissected sharply. Soft tissue dissection is done from the floor of the sinus tarsi to preserve the blood supply to the talar body. With this approach, reduction of the talar body with respect to the subtalar joint, alignment of the lateral talar neck, and reduction of the lateral process can be controlled.

Application of a femoral distractor is extremely helpful in exposing the surfaces of the subtalar joint. The pins are inserted into the medial aspect of the tibial shaft and the posterior aspect of the calcaneal tuberosity. Manipulation of the main talar head and body fragments is eased using joystick K-wires, which are introduced from medially.[31] The fractures are cleared from intervening soft tissue and comminuted fragments. After reduction of the talar neck and body from medial, anatomic reduction and congruity of the subtalar joint are checked from lateral.

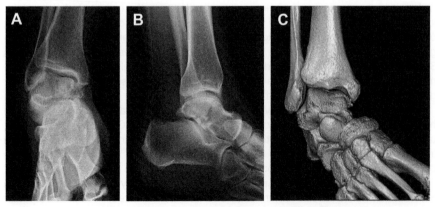

Fig. 3. (*A–C*) Rare combination of a central talar fracture and a subtalar dislocation.

Depending on the size and location of the fractured fragments at the talar body, the fractures are fixed with conventional or headless screws or small plates along the talar neck. Smaller chondral or osteochondral fragments are fixed with resorbable pins and fibrin glue or removed if not amenable to fixation. Rarely, lost K-wires may be used for small intermediate fragments containing firm subchondral bone (**Fig. 4**).

Fractures of the posterior talar body

Fractures of the posterior talar body involve both the ankle and subtalar joints. They are best visualized from a posterolateral approach to the ankle and subtalar joint with the patient prone or in a lateral decubitus position.[31] The longitudinal incision lies halfway between the lateral aspect of the Achilles tendon and the peroneal tendons.

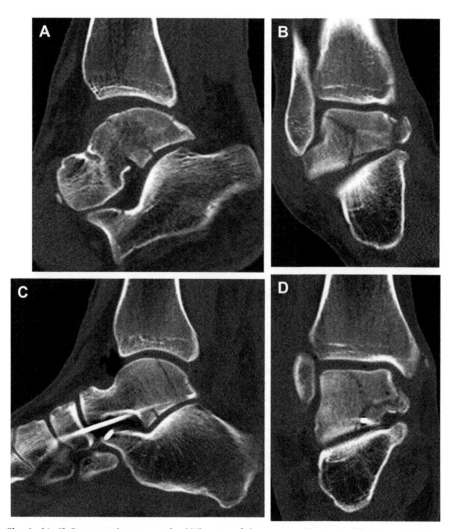

Fig. 4. (*A, B*) Computed tomography (CT) scans of the same patient as in **Fig. 2** on admission reveals a frontal fracture through the talar body with displaced fragments at the lateral aspect of the subtalar joint and the medial wall. (*C, D*) CT scans after open reduction via bilateral approaches and K-wire fixation show anatomic reconstruction of the subtalar joint.

The superficial and deep fascia is incised. The flexor hallucis longus muscle and tendon are held away to protect the posterior tibial neurovascular bundle. After resecting the posterior capsule, the ankle and subtalar joints are visualized. If the fracture extends far into the dorsomedial part of the talar body, a posteromedial approach is preferable.[3] The incision lies parallel to the medial aspect of the Achilles tendon. Preparation is carried out strictly lateral to the flexor hallucis longus tendon to protect the posteromedial neurovascular bundle. The deltoid ligament must not be dissected to avoid impairing the blood supply to the posterior talar body. Again, exposure of both joint surfaces can be improved with the application of a femoral distractor spanned between the calcaneus and the tibia. The posterior talar body is reduced and fixed under direct vision with small fragment screws (2.4–3.5 mm diameter, depending on the fragment size) or a small plate.[31,47]

Primary fusion of the subtalar joint should be considered only in cases of comminuted fractures with destruction of the articular surface.[46,48] The talonavicular joint as part of the coxa pedis should be preserved whenever possible.[40]

Results and complications

The functional results after talar fractures depend on the severity of the injury and the quality of reduction. Nonoperative treatment or inadequate reduction and fixation of displaced talar fractures frequently lead to unsatisfying results with persisting pain, loss of motion, and arthritic changes.[6,27,49] Malunions of the talar neck and body with symptomatic arthritis are treated with realignment and fusion of arthritic joints.[50]

Given the mechanism of injury for central talar fractures, there is an inherent risk for the development of posttraumatic arthritis in both the ankle and subtalar joints. The rates that are reported in the literature vary considerably from 16% to 100% after talar neck and body fractures, which may be due to the lack of uniform criteria and great variety of fracture patterns.[51–56] Most studies did not find a clear association between fracture classification and the occurrence of posttraumatic arthritis.[52–54] Moreover, the rates of arthritis depend on the duration of follow-up; subtalar arthritis in particular deteriorates over time.[51,55,56]

However, only a portion of patients with radiographic signs of posttraumatic arthritis becomes clinically symptomatic. Therefore, the reported fusion rates are considerably lower than the arthritis rate and range between 3% and 20%. In contrast, malalignment of the talar head, neck, body, and processes is closely related to the development of posttraumatic arthritis.[6,26,27] In compliant patients with adequate bone stock and viable cartilage where malalignment has not yet led to symptomatic arthritis, a joint-preserving osteotomy may be considered together with functional rehabilitation.[57] Symptomatic arthritis of the subtalar joint not responding to conservative measures requires fusion with realignment of any residual deformities.[1,50]

The prevalence of AVN as provided in various studies ranges from 0% to 24% in Hawkins type I fractures, from 0% to 50% in Hawkins type II fractures, and from 33% to 100% in Hawkins type III and IV fractures.[40] Undisplaced talar body fractures (Marti type II fractures) are associated with AVN in 5% to 44%, whereas AVN in displaced talar body fractures (Marti types III and IV fractures) average about 50%.[3,39,40] Open talar neck and body fractures seem to bear an increased risk of AVN in some studies,[51,53,54] although others did not confirm this association.[31,46] From a historical perspective, a more aggressive approach using early, stable internal fixation and functional postoperative protocol was able to considerably lower the rate of AVN of the talus as compared with earlier studies.[49,58]

CALCANEAL FRACTURES WITH SUBTALAR JOINT INVOLVEMENT
Etiology

The majority of calcaneal fractures are produced by axial forces like falls from height or in motor vehicle accidents. More than 75% of all calcaneal fractures are intraarticular and the largest joint facet, the convex posterior facet of the subtalar joint, is involved in almost 90% of all intraarticular calcaneal fractures.[59] In more than 50%, there is also involvement of the calcaneocuboid joint.[59]

The vertical axis of the calcaneus lies laterally to that of the talus. Therefore, with axial loading, the sustentaculum tali is sheared off the main body of the calcaneus, which bears the posterior facet of the subtalar joint. Consequently, the primary sagittal fracture line runs through the calcaneus and mostly through the subtalar joint.[60] In cases of fracture-dislocations, the whole calcaneal tuberosity is displaced laterally and toward the fibular tip, frequently producing an irregular distal fibular fracture with avulsion of the superior peroneal retinacle.[3,59] These injuries are frequently overlooked or misinterpreted as distal fibular fractures because they do not display the typical features of calcaneal fractures as outlined elsewhere in this article.

The coronal fracture lines also follow reproducible patterns, beginning (or exiting) at Gissane's angle and the posterior aspect of the subtalar joint.[61] In joint depression type fractures, a secondary fracture line exits behind the impacted posterior facet resulting in a depressed and tilted facet fragment. In tongue type fractures, the fracture exits through the superior part of the tuberosity, producing in a large fragment that is pulled upward by the Achilles tendon, giving it a tonguelike appearance.[62]

Diagnosis and Management

Clinical examination typically reveals pain, swelling, and hematoma at the hindfoot and the inability to bear weight. Deformities and axial deviations may be seen. Active or passive inversion and eversion of the foot is painful and the heel is tender to palpation. Blister formation may develop within a few hours and may indicate pressure from the inside by hematoma or displaced fragments. Repeated clinical examinations have been suggested to not overlook calcaneal fractures in polytraumatized or multiply injured patients after high-velocity trauma.[63]

Standard radiographs for a suspected calcaneal fracture include axial and lateral projections of the hindfoot. Anteroposterior radiographs of the ankle show the amount of calcaneofibular abutment and talar tilt in fracture-dislocations. If a displaced fracture is seen, lateral views of the unaffected calcaneus are useful to measure the individual normal values of Böhler's and Gissane's angles. Oblique views of the subtalar joint (Brodén series) that show the extent of damage to the subtalar joint are mainly used for intraoperative fluoroscopic control of joint reduction.[64] For any suspected intraarticular fracture a CT scan is needed for accurate analysis of the fracture morphology and to determine the treatment strategy (**Fig. 5**).

Subtalar joint dysfunction after malunited calcaneal fractures leads to a severely altered gait with pronounced difficulties and pain on uneven ground, ladders, and stairs.[1] Therefore, when operative treatment is chosen for displaced intraarticular calcaneal fractures, anatomic reduction of the subtalar joint is of utmost importance.[59,65–68] In biomechanical studies, even small step-offs of 1 to 2 mm in the posterior facet were associated with a considerable load transfers within the subtalar joint, increasing the risk of posttraumatic subtalar arthritis.[69,70] A multitude of clinical series has found inferior functional results in patients with residual incongruities within the subtalar joint.[71–76]

Failure to reduce the subtalar joint anatomically may be one reason why recent prospective randomized controlled trials (RCTs) did not find statistically significant

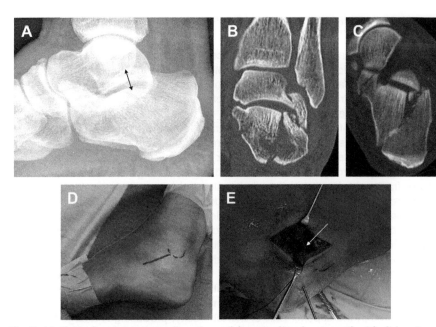

Fig. 5. (A–C) Displaced, intraarticular calcaneal fracture (Sanders type 3) with dislocation of the lateral joint fragment between the fibula and lateral facet of the talus and additional undisplaced fracture through the sustentaculum tali. Note the double contour over the subtalar joint and the overlap between talus and calcaneus (*double arrow in A*). (D, E) The subtalar joint is visualized via a sinus tarsi approach that is extended over the tip of the fibula to expose the dislocated joint fragment (*white arrow*).

differences between operative and nonoperative treatment for displaced intraarticular calcaneal fractures.[74,77,78] A close look at the results reveals that two of those studies demonstrated residual step-offs within the subtalar joint of 2 mm or more in 22% to 40% of the patients surgically treated.[77,78] In the third RCT, significantly better results were seen for patients with adequate joint reduction (within 2 mm)[74] and the same was observed in a post hoc analysis of another RCT.[79]

Two of these 3 recent RCTs found significantly higher rates of subtalar fusions for patients treated nonoperatively.[74,78] In the third RCT, secondary subtalar fusions were performed exclusively in the nonoperative group, although the difference was not statistically significant.[78] Consequently, anatomic reduction of intraarticular fractures with joint displacement of 2 mm and more is generally recommended.

Extensile lateral approach
Traditionally, the majority of displaced, intraarticular fractures have been treated effectively via an extensile lateral approach.[65] It allows good visualization of the posterior subtalar facet, the calcaneocuboid joint, and for restoration of the fractured lateral wall.

Direct manipulation of the tuberosity fragment with a Schanz screw introduced percutaneously is very useful for mobilizing the impacted intraarticular fragments and later reduction.[59,65] An important first step is reduction of the medial calcaneal wall by moving the tuberosity fragment plantarly and medially below the sustentacular fragment, carrying the medial facet of the subtalar joint. To achieve this, an elevator is introduced a lever between these 2 fragments.[80] The fragments are fixed to each other with 1 or 2 K-wires and reduction of the medial wall is controlled fluoroscopically. If the tuberosity fragment is not reduced adequately, articular reduction may not be possible and tilting of the main articular fragments will then result in persistent incongruities. If intermediate joint fragment(s) are present, these are then reduced and fixed to the sustentacular fragment with 1 or 2 K-wires that are pulled through the medial cortex and the skin medially so that they are flush with the intermediate fragment on the lateral side.[3,59] Small intermediate fragments with intact cartilage cover may alternatively be fixed with lost K-wires or absorbable pins.[81] Finally, the depressed lateral portion of the posterior facet is reduced to the medial fragment(s) using the inferior articular surface of the talus as a template and the K-wires are drilled back into this fragment from medial. If the lateral joint fragment is part of a tongue fragment extending to the posterior wall of the tuberosity, anatomic reduction of this fragment at the joint level sometimes is impossible because of soft tissue restraints. In these cases, an osteotomy behind the joint surface turning the tongue fracture into a joint depression fracture allows for exact reduction of the tilted posterior facet.[82]

The subtalar joint should be reduced anatomically. The quality of reduction of the subtalar joint should be checked either by open subtalar arthroscopy[83] or intraoperative 3-dimensional fluoroscopy.[84] This step is specifically important if the fracture is located far medially or with multiple fragmentation of the subtalar joint. The lateral aspect of the joint can be checked visually. If an intraarticular step-off is found, the position of the posterior facet can be corrected immediately, thus preventing painful postoperative conditions or the need for further surgery. Clinical studies have shown that arthroscopy and 3-dimensional fluoroscopy are able to show relevant irregularities or screw malpositioning within the subtalar joint that had not been detected clinically or by conventional fluoroscopy in more than 20% of cases.[83,84] After anatomic reduction of the joint is confirmed, the joint fragments are stabilized with 1 or 2 screws directed toward the sustentaculum.

The reconstructed subtalar joint block is then reduced to the tuberosity fragment. The heel height is restored and any varus or valgus deformity of the tuberosity is eliminated using the Schanz screw as a lever. Finally, the anterior process is reduced to the posterior part of the calcaneus and temporarily fixed with K-wires. Restoration of the outer shape of the calcaneus is controlled fluoroscopically. Definite fixation is achieved with a plate applied to the lateral wall and screws directed into the sustentaculum tali, the tuberosity, and the anterior process.[3,80]

Sinus tarsi approach

To minimize the wound healing problems and infections that are invariably associated with extensile approaches, less invasive or percutaneous fixation of calcaneal fractures have always been discussed as an alternative treatment.[85] Over the last decade, a small incision of 3 to 4 cm directly above the angle of Gissane (sinus tarsi approach) has gained increasing popularity.[86–90] This approach allows a good visualization of the posterior facet and reduction of the joint surface under direct vision (see **Fig. 5**). The peroneal tendons are identified, mobilized within their sheaths, and held away plantarly. The subtalar joint is accessed directly from the sinus tarsi and cleared of hematoma and small debris. The sequence of reduction is the same as with an extensile lateral approach.[88] A smooth elevator is introduced gently into the primary fracture line between the sustentaculum and the tuberosity fragments and used as a lever to align the medial wall and bring the tuberosity fragment beneath the sustentaculum. The main fragments are manipulated percutaneously as described elsewhere in this article, but the joint fragments can be manipulated directly through this approach. With multiple fragmentation of the posterior facet, the additional use of dry arthroscopy for precise control of joint reduction may be useful (**Fig. 6**).

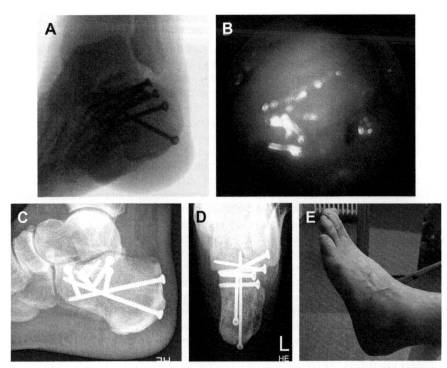

Fig. 6. (*A*) The posterior facet of the subtalar joint is reduced from medial to lateral. (*B*) Anatomic reduction of the 2 fracture lines is controlled with open (dry) subtalar arthroscopy. (*C, D*) Radiographs at 8 weeks follow-up show bony consolidation. (*E*) The scar from the sinus tarsi approach has healed uneventfully (same patient as in **Fig. 5**).

Definite fixation is achieved with percutaneous screws or bolts, an intramedullary nail with locking screws, or a small plate that is slid in through the approach and tunneled beneath the peroneal tendons.[86–92] Recent comparative studies show reduced rates of soft tissue complications while achieving and maintaining adequate reduction.[89,92]

In selected patients, entirely percutaneous reduction and fixation may be feasible. Because percutaneous fixation carries the risk of inadequate reduction of the subtalar joint, this technique is most suitable in extraarticular and simple intraarticular fractures (Sanders type II fractures).[93,94] Anatomic joint reduction should be controlled by subtalar arthroscopy.[85,94–96]

Fracture-dislocations of the calcaneus

Fracture-dislocations of the calcaneus are rare but often misjudged injuries with wide separation between the sustentacular fragment and the whole calcaneal body carrying the tuberosity and most of the subtalar joint (**Fig. 7**). The superolateral dislocation of the calcaneal body results in a direct compression of the fibular tip with subsequent dislocation of the peroneal tendons.[97] Sometimes, a distal fibular fracture is seen that may be mistaken for a malleolar fracture.[50] In the lateral view, there is a characteristic double density because of an overlap of the contours of the talus and calcaneus. Otherwise, the overall shape of the calcaneus seems to remain intact. However, in an anteroposterior view of the ankle, the direct fibulocalcaneal impingement (abutment) is seen and often the wide gap in the subtalar joint can be visualized directly.

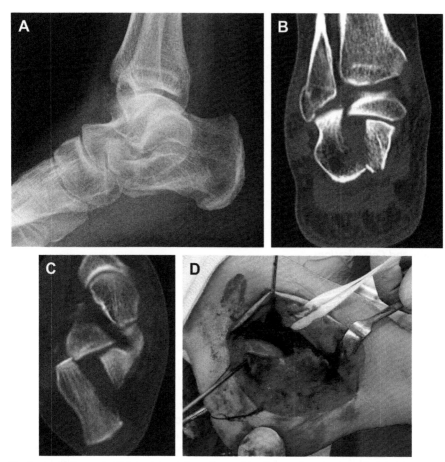

Fig. 7. (*A–C*) Fracture-dislocation of the calcaneal body carrying the lateral part of the subtalar joint beneath the fibular tip. Computed tomography scans show the wide separation of the main fragments. (*D*) Open reduction is carried out via a lateral approach starting over the fibular tip and extending toward the anterior process depending on the fracture morphology. The dislocated peroneal tendons are held aside. (*E*) The main fragments are reduced with a curved reduction clamp placed on the sustentaculum tali and the lateral wall and the fracture is stabilized with compression screws. (*F, G*) Anteroposterior and lateral radiographs at 3 months showing bony union.

Calcaneal fracture-dislocations should be reduced early via an extension of the sinus tarsi approach (dislocation approach according to Zwipp and colleagues[59]). It starts over the lateral malleolus and allows access to the displaced tuberosity and lateral joint fragment from above. When dissecting the subcutaneous tissue, care must be taken not to injure the peroneal tendons, which are invariably dislocated lateral to and above the tip of the fibula.[88] If performed early, reduction of the calcaneal body to the sustentaculum is rather straightforward and joint reduction can be judged under direct vision. Fracture fixation is mainly achieved with lag screws across the primary fracture line and directed into the sustentaculum.[80] An accompanying fibular fracture is fixed with minifragment screws, the peroneal tendons are rerouted into the fibular groove and the superior peroneal retinacle is sutured or reattached.[59,88]

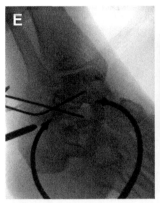 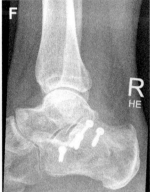 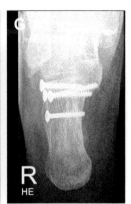

Fig. 7. (*continued*).

Results and Complications

A multitude of clinical studies reports the short- to mid-term results after various treatment protocols for intraarticular calcaneal fractures. Large clinical series with more than 100 patients who were followed for more than 1 year showed good to excellent results with open reduction and lateral plate fixation in 60% to 85% of cases using different outcome criteria.[67,71,80,98] These results seem to prevail over time in series with 8 to 15 years of follow-up.[76,99–101] These and other studies also have identified several patient-related negative prognostic factors that include severity of the fracture pattern, open and bilateral fractures, eligibility for workers' compensation, and high workload.[74,76,101–103]

Operative treatment of displaced, intraarticular fractures is challenging both with respect to adequate reduction and soft tissue handling. It is, therefore, associated with a considerable learning curve for the individual surgeon.[67,103] Consequently, higher complication rates and less favorable outcomes are observed in studies with a lower caseload.[104] Reconstruction of hindfoot geometry as measured by Böhler's angle has been identified as a positive prognostic factor that may be influenced by the surgeon.[75,102,105,106] However, reconstruction of the subtalar joint remains one of the most important goals in calcaneal fracture surgery. Numerous clinical studies have shown that failure to reduce the posterior facet of the subtalar joint within 2 mm results in significantly inferior outcomes.[71–75,107,108]

Beside subtalar arthritis, which may potentially be minimized but not completely avoided with anatomic joint reconstruction, wound complications and infections remain a concern with operative treatment of calcaneal fractures. With the use of minimally invasive approaches, the rates of wound complications and infections requiring operative revision could be lowered substantially, although similar reduction rates could be observed.[86–92] Given the importance of anatomic joint reduction of the subtalar joint for postoperative foot function, less invasive or percutaneous approaches should not be used at the cost of less than optimal joint reconstruction.[85,94]

REFERENCES

1. Rammelt S, Grass R, Zawadski T, et al. Foot function after subtalar distraction bone-block arthrodesis. A prospective study. J Bone Joint Surg Br 2004; 86(5):659–68.
2. Greiner TM. The jargon of pedal movements. Foot Ankle Int 2007;28(1):109–25.

3. Zwipp H, Rammelt S. Tscherne Unfallchirurgie. Fuss. Berlin: Springer; 2014.
4. De Wulf A. Anatomic macro- et microscopique du sinus du tarse. Chir Piede 1980;4:1.
5. Rammelt S, Goronzy J. Subtalar dislocations. Foot Ankle Clin 2015;20(2): 253–64.
6. Rammelt S, Winkler J, Grass R, et al. Reconstruction after talar fractures. Foot Ankle Clin 2006;11(1):61–84, viii.
7. Ball ST, Jadin K, Allen RT, et al. Chondrocyte viability after intra-articular calcaneal fractures in humans. Foot Ankle Int 2007;28(6):665–8.
8. Bibbo C, Anderson RB, Davis WH. Injury characteristics and the clinical outcome of subtalar dislocations: a clinical and radiographic analysis of 25 cases. Foot Ankle Int 2003;24(2):158–63.
9. Gregory P, DiPasquale T, Herscovici D, et al. Ipsilateral fractures of the talus and calcaneus. Foot Ankle Int 1996;17(11):701–5.
10. Seybold D, Schildhauer TA, Muhr G. Combined ipsilateral fractures of talus and calcaneus. Foot Ankle Int 2008;29(3):318–24.
11. Aminian A, Howe CR, Sangeorzan BJ, et al. Ipsilateral talar and calcaneal fractures: a retrospective review of complications and sequelae. Injury 2009;40(2): 139–45.
12. Zimmer TJ, Johnson KA. Subtalar dislocations. Clin Orthop Rel Res 1989;(238): 190–4.
13. de Palma L, Santucci A, Marinelli M, et al. Clinical outcome of closed isolated subtalar dislocations. Arch Orthop Trauma Surg 2008;128(6):593–8.
14. Goldner JL, Poletti SC, Gates HS 3rd, et al. Severe open subtalar dislocations. Long-term results. J Bone Joint Surg Am 1995;77(7):1075–9.
15. Bibbo C, Lin SS, Abidi N, et al. Missed and associated injuries after subtalar dislocation: the role of CT. Foot Ankle Int 2001;22(4):324–8.
16. Buckingham WW Jr, LeFlore I. Subtalar dislocation of the foot. J Trauma 1973; 13(9):753–65.
17. Grantham SA. Medial subtalar dislocation: five cases with a common etiology. J Trauma 1964;4:845–9.
18. Hoexum F, Heetveld MJ. Subtalar dislocation: two cases requiring surgery and a literature review of the last 25 years. Arch Orthop Trauma Surg 2014;134(9): 1237–49.
19. Leitner B. Behandlungen und Behandlungsergebnisse von 42 frischen Fällen von Luxatio pedis sub talo im Unfallkrankenhaus Wien. Ergebnisse Chir Orthop 1952;37:501–77.
20. Inokuchi S, Hashimoto T, Usami N. Anterior subtalar dislocation: case report. J Orthop Trauma 1997;11(3):235–7.
21. Inokuchi S, Hashimoto T, Usami N. Posterior subtalar dislocation. J Trauma 1997;42(2):310–3.
22. Rammelt S, Schepers T. Chopart injuries: when to fix and when to fuse? Foot Ankle Clin 2017;22(1):163–80.
23. Main BJ, Jowett RL. Injuries of the midtarsal joint. J Bone Joint Surg Br 1975; 57(1):89–97.
24. Bohay DR, Manoli A 2nd. Occult fractures following subtalar joint injuries. Foot Ankle Int 1996;17(3):164–9.
25. Dürr C, Zwipp H, Rammelt S. Fractures of the sustentaculum tali. Oper Orthop Traumatol 2013;25(6):569–78.
26. Lorentzen JE, Christensen SB, Krogsoe O, et al. Fractures of the neck of the talus. Acta Orthop Scand 1977;48(1):115–20.

27. Sneppen O, Christensen SB, Krogsoe O, et al. Fracture of the body of the talus. Acta Orthop Scand 1977;48(3):317–24.
28. Giuffrida AY, Lin SS, Abidi N, et al. Pseudo os trigonum sign: missed posteromedial talar facet fracture. Foot Ankle Int 2003;24(8):642–9.
29. Langer P, Nickisch F, Spenciner D, et al. Effect of simulated lateral process talus "fracture excision" on its ligamentous attachments. Am J Orthop 2009;38(5):222–6.
30. Rammelt S, Zwipp H, Prescher A. Talus bipartitus: a rare skeletal variation: a report of four cases. J Bone Joint Surg Am 2011;93(6):e21.
31. Rammelt S, Winkler J, Zwipp H. Operative treatment of central talar fractures. Oper Orthop Traumatol 2013;25(6):525–41 [in German].
32. Cronier P, Talha A, Massin P. Central talar fractures–therapeutic considerations. Injury 2004;35(Suppl 2):SB10–22.
33. Della Rocca GJ, Nork SE, Barei DP, et al. Fractures of the sustentaculum tali: injury characteristics and surgical technique for reduction. Foot Ankle Int 2009;30(11):1037–41.
34. Merchan EC. Subtalar dislocations: long-term follow-up of 39 cases. Injury 1992;23(2):97–100.
35. Milenkovic S, Mitkovic M, Bumbasirevic M. External fixation of open subtalar dislocation. Injury 2006;37(9):909–13.
36. Jungbluth P, Wild M, Hakimi M, et al. Isolated subtalar dislocation. J Bone Joint Surg Am 2010;92(4):890–4.
37. Heppenstall RB, Farahvar H, Balderston R, et al. Evaluation and management of subtalar dislocations. J Trauma 1980;20(6):494–7.
38. Assal M, Stern R. Total extrusion of the talus. A case report. J Bone Joint Surg Am 2004;86-A(12):2726–31.
39. Marti R. Talus und Calcaneusfrakturen. In: Weber BG, Brunner C, Freuler F, editors. Die Frakturenbehandlung bei Kindern und Jugendlichen. Berlin: Springer-Verlag; 1974. p. 376–87.
40. Rammelt S, Zwipp H. Talar neck and body fractures. Injury 2009;40(2):120–35.
41. Daniels TR, Smith JW, Ross TI. Varus malalignment of the talar neck. Its effect on the position of the foot and on subtalar motion. J Bone Joint Surg Am 1996;78(10):1559–67.
42. Fortin PT, Balazsy JE. Talus fractures: evaluation and treatment. J Am Acad Orthop Surg 2001;9(2):114–27.
43. Juliano PJ, Dabbah M, Harris TG. Talar neck fractures. Foot Ankle Clin 2004;9(4):723–36, vi.
44. Thordarson DB. Talar body fractures. Orthop Clin North Am 2001;32(1):65–77, viii.
45. Inokuchi S, Ogawa K, Usami N. Classification of fractures of the talus: clear differentiation between neck and body fractures. Foot Ankle Int 1996;17(12):748–50.
46. Schulze W, Richter J, Russe O, et al. Surgical treatment of talus fractures: a retrospective study of 80 cases followed for 1-15 years. Acta Orthop Scand 2002;73(3):344–51.
47. Shank JR, Benirschke SK, Swords MP. Treatment of peripheral talus fractures. Foot Ankle Clin 2017;22(1):181–92.
48. Thomas RH, Daniels TR. Primary fusion as salvage following talar neck fracture: a case report. Foot Ankle Int 2003;24(4):368–71.
49. Canale ST, Kelly FB Jr. Fractures of the neck of the talus. J Bone Joint Surg Am 1978;60:143–56.

50. Rammelt S, Zwipp H. Corrective arthrodeses and osteotomies for post-traumatic hindfoot malalignment: indications, techniques, results. Int Orthop 2013;37(9): 1707–17.
51. Lindvall E, Haidukewych G, DiPasquale T, et al. Open reduction and stable fixation of isolated, displaced talar neck and body fractures. J Bone Joint Surg Am 2004;86-A(10):2229–34.
52. Schuind F, Andrianne Y, Burny F, et al. Fractures et luxations de l'astragale. Revue de 359 cas. Acta Orthop Belg 1983;49(6):652–89.
53. Vallier HA, Nork SE, Barei DP, et al. Talar neck fractures: results and outcomes. J Bone Joint Surg Am 2004;86-A(8):1616–24.
54. Vallier HA, Nork SE, Benirschke SK, et al. Surgical treatment of talar body fractures. J Bone Joint Surg Am 2003;85-A(9):1716–24.
55. Ohl X, Harisboure A, Hemery X, et al. Long-term follow-up after surgical treatment of talar fractures: twenty cases with an average follow-up of 7.5 years. Int Orthop 2011;35(1):93–9.
56. Sanders DW, Busam M, Hattwick E, et al. Functional outcomes following displaced talar neck fractures. J Orthop Trauma 2004;18(5):265–70.
57. Rammelt S, Winkler J, Heineck J, et al. Anatomical reconstruction of malunited talus fractures: a prospective study of 10 patients followed for 4 years. Acta Orthop 2005;76(4):588–96.
58. Hawkins LG. Fractures of the neck of the talus. J Bone Joint Surg Am 1970; 52(5):991–1002.
59. Zwipp H, Rammelt S, Barthel S. Calcaneal fractures–open reduction and internal fixation (ORIF). Injury 2004;35(Suppl 2):SB46–54.
60. Miric A, Patterson BM. Pathoanatomy of intra-articular fractures of the calcaneus. J Bone Joint Surg Am 1998;80(2):207–12.
61. Carr JB. Mechanism and pathoanatomy of the intraarticular calcaneal fracture. Clin Orthop Rel Res 1993;(290):36–40.
62. Essex-Lopresti P. The mechanism, reduction technique, and results in fractures of the os calcis. Br J Surg 1952;39:395–419.
63. Rammelt S, Biewener A, Grass R, et al. Foot injuries in the polytraumatized patient. Unfallchirurg 2005;108(10):858–65 [in German].
64. Brodén B. Roentgen examination of the subtaloid joint in fractures of the calcaneus. Acta Radiol 1949;31:85–8.
65. Benirschke SK, Sangeorzan BJ. Extensive intraarticular fractures of the foot. Surgical management of calcaneal fractures. Clin Orthop Relat Res 1993;(292):128–34.
66. Crosby LA, Fitzgibbons T. Intraarticular calcaneal fractures. Results of closed treatment. Clin Orthop Rel Res 1993;(290):47–54.
67. Zwipp H, Tscherne H, Thermann H, et al. Osteosynthesis of displaced intraarticular fractures of the calcaneus. Results in 123 cases. Clin Orthop Rel Res 1993;(290):76–86.
68. Sanders R. Displaced intra-articular fractures of the calcaneus. J Bone Joint Surg Am 2000;82(2):225–50.
69. Sangeorzan BJ, Ananthakrishnan D, Tencer AF. Contact characteristics of the subtalar joint after a simulated calcaneus fracture. J Orthop Trauma 1995; 9(3):251–8.
70. Mulcahy DM, McCormack DM, Stephens MM. Intra-articular calcaneal fractures: effect of open reduction and internal fixation on the contact characteristics of the subtalar joint. Foot Ankle Int 1998;19(12):842–8.

71. Brattebø J, Mølster AO, Wirsching J. Fractures of the calcaneus: a retrospective study of 115 fractures. Ortho Int 1995;3:117 26.

72. Song KS, Kang CH, Min BW, et al. Preoperative and postoperative evaluation of intra-articular fractures of the calcaneus based on computed tomography scanning. J Orthop Trauma 1997;11(6):435–40.

73. Boack DH, Wichelhaus A, Mittlmeier T, et al. Therapy of dislocated calcaneus joint fracture with the AO calcaneus plate. Chirurg 1998;69(11):1214–23 [in German].

74. Buckley R, Tough S, McCormack R, et al. Operative compared with nonoperative treatment of displaced intra- articular calcaneal fractures: a prospective, randomized, controlled multicenter trial. J Bone Joint Surg Am 2002;84-A(10): 1733–44.

75. Rammelt S, Barthel S, Biewener A, et al. Calcaneus fractures. Open reduction and internal fixation. Zentralbl Chir 2003;128:517–28 [in German].

76. Rammelt S, Zwipp H, Schneiders W, et al. Severity of injury predicts subsequent function in surgically treated displaced intraarticular calcaneal fractures. Clin Orthop Rel Res 2013;471(9):2885–98.

77. Agren PH, Wretenberg P, Sayed-Noor AS. Operative versus nonoperative treatment of displaced intra-articular calcaneal fractures: a prospective, randomized, controlled multicenter trial. J Bone Joint Surg Am 2013;95(15):1351–7.

78. Griffin D, Parsons N, Shaw E, et al. Operative versus non-operative treatment for closed, displaced, intra-articular fractures of the calcaneus: randomised controlled trial. Br Med J 2014;349:g4483.

79. Agren PH, Mukka S, Tullberg T, et al. Factors affecting long-term treatment results of displaced intraarticular calcaneal fractures: a post hoc analysis of a prospective, randomized, controlled multicenter trial. J Orthop Trauma 2014;28(10): 564–8.

80. Sanders R, Rammelt S. Fractures of the calcaneus. In: Coughlin MJ, Saltzman CR, Anderson JB, editors. Mann's surgery of the foot & ankle. 9th edition. St Louis (MO): Elsevier; 2013. p. 2041–100.

81. Min W, Munro M, Sanders R. Stabilization of displaced articular fragments in calcaneal fractures using bioabsorbable pin fixation: a technique guide. J Orthop Trauma 2010;24(12):770–4.

82. Sanders R. Turning tongues into joint depressions: a new calcaneal osteotomy. J Orthop Trauma 2012;26(3):193–6.

83. Rammelt S, Gavlik JM, Barthel S, et al. The value of subtalar arthroscopy in the management of intra-articular calcaneus fractures. Foot Ankle Int 2002;23(10): 906–16.

84. Rubberdt A, Feil R, Stengel D, et al. The clinical use of the ISO-C(3D) imaging system in calcaneus fracture surgery. Unfallchirurg 2006;109(2):112–8 [in German].

85. Rammelt S, Amlang M, Barthel S, et al. Minimally-invasive treatment of calcaneal fractures. Injury 2004;35(Suppl 2):SB55–63.

86. Weber M, Lehmann O, Sagesser D, et al. Limited open reduction and internal fixation of displaced intra-articular fractures of the calcaneum. J Bone Joint Surg Br 2008;90(12):1608–16.

87. Nosewicz T, Knupp M, Barg A, et al. Mini-open sinus tarsi approach with percutaneous screw fixation of displaced calcaneal fractures: a prospective computed tomography-based study. Foot Ankle Int 2012;33(11):925–33.

88. Rammelt S, Zwipp H. Fractures of the calcaneus: current treatment strategies. Acta Chir Orthop Traumatol Cech 2014;81(3):177–96.

89. Schepers T, Backes M, Dingemans SA, et al. Similar anatomical reduction and lower complication rates with the sinus tarsi approach compared with the extended lateral approach in displaced intra-articular calcaneal fractures. J Orthop Trauma 2017;31(6):293–8.

90. Zwipp H, Pasa L, Zilka L, et al. Introduction of a new locking nail for treatment of intraarticular calcaneal fractures. J Orthop Trauma 2016;30(3):e88–92.

91. Goldzak M, Mittlmeier T, Simon P. Locked nailing for the treatment of displaced articular fractures of the calcaneus: description of a new procedure with calcanail((R)). Eur J Orthop Surg Traumatol 2012;22(4):345–9.

92. Kline AJ, Anderson RB, Davis WH, et al. Minimally invasive technique versus an extensile lateral approach for intra-articular calcaneal fractures. Foot Ankle Int 2013;34(6):773–80.

93. Tornetta P 3rd. The Essex-Lopresti reduction for calcaneal fractures revisited. J Orthop Trauma 1998;12(7):469–73.

94. Rammelt S, Amlang M, Barthel S, et al. Percutaneous treatment of less severe intraarticular calcaneal fractures. Clin Orthop Rel Res 2010;468(4):983–90.

95. Woon CY, Chong KW, Yeo W, et al. Subtalar arthroscopy and fluoroscopy in percutaneous fixation of intra-articular calcaneal fractures: the best of both worlds. J Trauma 2011;71(4):917–25.

96. Yeap EJ, Rao J, Pan CH, et al. Is arthroscopic assisted percutaneous screw fixation as good as open reduction and internal fixation for the treatment of displaced intra-articular calcaneal fractures? Foot Ankle Surg 2016;22(3):164–9.

97. Court-Brown CM, Boot DA, Kellam JF. Fracture dislocation of the calcaneus. A report of two cases. Clin Orthop Rel Res 1986;(213):201–6.

98. Letournel E. Open treatment of acute calcaneal fractures. Clin Orthop Rel Res 1993;(290):60–7.

99. Potter MQ, Nunley JA. Long-term functional outcomes after operative treatment for intra-articular fractures of the calcaneus. J Bone Joint Surg Am 2009;91(8):1854–60.

100. Rammelt S. An update on the treatment of calcaneal fractures. J Orthop Trauma 2014;28(10):549–50.

101. Sanders R, Vaupel Z, Erdogan M, et al. Operative treatment of displaced intra-articular calcaneal fractures: long-term (10-20 years) results in 108 fractures using a prognostic CT classification. J Orthop Trauma 2014;28(10):551–63.

102. Paley D, Hall H. Intra-articular fractures of the calcaneus. A critical analysis of results and prognostic factors. J Bone Joint Surg Am 1993;75(3):342–54.

103. Sanders R, Fortin P, DiPasquale A, et al. The results of operative treatment of displaced intra-articular calcaneal fractures using a CT scan classification. In: Tscherne H, Schatzker J, editors. Major fractures of the pilon, the talus and the calcaneus. Berlin: Springer Verlag; 1992. p. 175–89.

104. Poeze M, Verbruggen JP, Brink PR. The relationship between the outcome of operatively treated calcaneal fractures and institutional fracture load. A systematic review of the literature. J Bone Joint Surg Am 2008;90(5):1013–21.

105. Paul M, Peter R, Hoffmeyer P. Fractures of the calcaneum. A review of 70 patients. J Bone Joint Surg Br 2004;86(8):1142–5.

106. Makki D, Alnajjar HM, Walkay S, et al. Osteosynthesis of displaced intra-articular fractures of the calcaneum: a long-term review of 47 cases. J Bone Joint Surg Br 2010;92(5):693–700.

107. Janzen DL, Connell DG, Munk PL, et al. Intraarticular fractures of the calcaneus: value of CT findings in determining prognosis. AJR Am J Roentgenol 1992;158(6):1271–4.

108. van Hoeve S, de Vos J, Verbruggen JP, et al. Gait analysis and functional outcome after calcaneal fracture. J Bone Joint Surg Am 2015;97(22):1879–88.
109. Ruiz Valdivieso T, de Miguel Vielba JA, Hernandez Garcia C, et al. Subtalar dislocation. A study of nineteen cases. Int Orthop 1996;20(2):83–6.
110. Ruhlmann F, Poujardieu C, Vernois J, et al. Isolated acute traumatic subtalar dislocations: review of 13 cases at a mean follow-up of 6 years and literature review. J Foot Ankle Surg 2017;56(1):201–7.
111. Isay M, Wolvius R, Ochsner PE. Long-term results of talus fractures. Z Unfallchir Versicherungsmed 1992;85(1):12–8 [in German].
112. Lutz M, Golser K, Sperner G, et al. Post-traumatic ischemia of the talus. Is talus necrosis unavoidable? Unfallchirurg 1998;101(6):461–7 [in German].
113. Elgafy H, Ebraheim NA, Tile M, et al. Fractures of the talus: experience of two level 1 trauma centers. Foot Ankle Int 2000;21(12):1023–9.
114. Ebraheim NA, Patil V, Owens C, et al. Clinical outcome of fractures of the talar body. Int Orthop 2008;32(6):773–7.
115. Fournier A, Barba N, Steiger V, et al. Total talar fracture - long-term results of internal fixation of talar fractures. A multicentric study of 114 cases. Orthop Traumatol Surg Res 2012;98(4 Suppl):S48–55.
116. Tantavisut S, Phisitkul P, Westerlind BO, et al. Percutaneous reduction and screw fixation of displaced intra-articular fractures of the calcaneus. Foot Ankle Int 2017;38(4):367–74.

Fractures of the Lateral Process of the Talus

Christian Tinner, MD, Christoph Sommer, MD*

KEYWORDS

- Talus • Ankle • LTPF • Lateral talar process fracture • Snowboarder's ankle
- New fracture classification of LTPF • ORIF talar fracture

KEY POINTS

- Lateral talar process fractures (LTPFs) are uncommon injuries but have become more relevant with snowboarding.
- Most fractures require surgical treatment following the principles of open reduction and internal fixation of displaced articular fractures.
- Stable fixation is achieved with small screws and often, if multifragmented, with small T-plates in buttress function.
- Associated injuries, like other foot fractures and/or peroneal tendon dislocation, are common and must be addressed at the same time.
- Overall prognosis is good, but long-term problems may develop and rarely require further surgical procedures.

 Video content accompanies this article at http://www.foot.theclinics.com/.

INTRODUCTION AND EPIDEMIOLOGY

Fractures of the lateral process of the talus (LTPFs) are uncommon injuries. Of all fractures, 0.1% to 0.85% are talar fractures and only 20% of these concern the LTPF.[1] With increased popularity of snowboarding sport, the incidence of this fracture has continuously raised.[2–5] The literature reveals that 15% of snowboarders ankle injuries are correlated with LTPFs. That means that this kind of fracture accounts for 2.3% of all snowboarding injuries.[6] The symptoms of an LTPF are similar to those of an ankle sprain and explains the frequent overlook and misdiagnosis of this fracture.[7] Once missed, it can result in significant sequels, including malunion, nonunion and degeneration of the subtalar joint.[8]

Disclosure: The authors have nothing to disclose.
Departement of Surgery, Kantonsspital Graubünden, Loëstrasse 170, Chur 7000, Switzerland
* Corresponding author.
E-mail address: christoph.sommer@ksgr.ch

Within the period from 2001 to 2017, the database (open reduction and internal fixation [ORIF]) of the authors' hospital demonstrated 55 patients who needed an ORIF for LTPF. Most of them, 38% (21 patients), had a snowboarding accident, 14% (8 patients) had a climbing accident, and 9% a car accident. All other patients sustained an injury at work, on motorbikes, as pedestrians, or during other sports activities.

Most of the LTPFs were isolated fractures (48 patients [87%]). Only 10% had additional ipsilateral foot fractures (6 patients talar neck and 1 patient anterior process of the talus).

In the same period, the authors operated on exactly the same number of other talar fractures (55 patients) without LTPF; most of them involved the talar neck (28 patients [51%]), followed by the talar body (10 patients [18%]) and other talar fractures (17 patients [31%]).

The incidence of LTPF caused by snowboard injuries alone has decreased remarkably in the past ten years. Analyzing the authors' figures in a 6-year period, the number of ORIFs for LTPFs has decreased from 22 cases (1995–2001) to 10 cases (2002–2008) to only 5 cases (2009–2014). From 2015 to 2017, there was only 1 snowboarder requiring surgical treatment. The authors assume 2 reasons for this change: on one hand, snowboarding has lost popularity, and on the other hand, what might be more important, the progress in development of shoes and bindings has led to a better overall protection of foot structures.

MECHANISM OF INJURY

There have been lot of discussions regarding the exact mechanism causing a LTPF.[9] Hawkins stated that the fracture is produced by forced dorsiflexion of the foot with associated inversion.[10] Other investigators showed evidence from in vitro biomechanical and clinical studies, suggesting that dorsiflexion, axial impaction, eversion, and external rotation are involved.[11] The authors believe that different mechanisms are possible. In the authors' opinion, it seems logical that the mechanism in a car accident might not be the same as a twist of the ankle in a snowboard boot or when landing after a climbing fall. The fracture patterns also differ from single small or large fragments to completely comminuted fractures, indicating the variability of fracture mechanisms.

CLASSIFICATION
Old Classifications

According to Hawkins, 3 types of LTPF are classified. First are the simple fractures that extend from the talofibular articular surface down to the posterior talocalcaneal articular surface of the subtalar joint. Second are the comminuted fractures that involve both the fibular and the posterior calcaneal articular surfaces of the talus and the entire lateral process. And third are chip fractures of the anterior and inferior portion of the posterior articular process of the talus; this type does not extend to the talofibular articulation.[10]

McCrory and Bladin,[12] as well as other investigators, reorganized Hawkins' original classification in an attempt to better guide treatment regimens. According to their categorization, type I is a nonarticular chip fracture, type II is a single large fragment involving the talofibular articulation and subtalar joint, and type III is a comminuted fracture also involving both articulations. The McCrory-Bladin classification is actually the most used classification of this fracture[12] (**Fig. 1**).

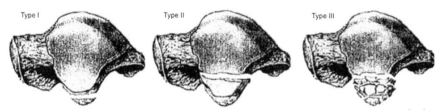

Fig. 1. McCrory-Bladin classification of LTPF. Type I, chip fractures; type II, simple fracture, large fragment; and type III, multifragmentary. (*From* McCrory P, Bladin C. Fractures of the lateral process of the talus: a clinical review. "Snowboarder's Ankle". Clin J Sport Med 1996;6:124–8; with permission.)

Proposal of a Newly Modified Classification

Concerning the existing classification, type I is rare in the authors' collective but does exist (~5% of all LTPFs). Larger isolated fragments (true type II) are also rare, because most of these larger fragment fractures are associated with 1 or more intermediate articular fragment of the subtalar facet and, therefore, are not single fragment fractures. But, because most of these fractures are not comminuted, they cannot really be classified according to the Bladin-McCrory classification. Finally, the multifragmentary type III, as shown in **Fig. 1**, is also rare.

The authors suggest modifying the existing classification slightly (**Fig. 2**); type I and type II remain the same, but type III is divided into 3 subtypes, IIIa, IIIb, and IIIc. This change of the classification has a direct influence on the operative treatment, especially the reduction and choice of implants. This is explained later.

In addition to the fracture classification, all fractures are assessed for their displacement: the authors distinguish no (or minimal) displaced fractures (<1 mm articular step, <2-mm gap) from displaced fractures (≥1-mm articular step, ≥2-mm gap). In the authors' experience, a majority of the fractures are displaced.

ASSOCIATED INJURIES

Most of the LTPFs are isolated fractures and only rarely are other additional fractures detected, such as of the talus (neck or anterior process), the calcaneus (posterior facet or sustentaculum), or other parts of the foot. In most cases, however, other significant associated hindfoot injuries are detected either clinically, on CT (or MRI), or during the operation.[13] These include calcaneal cartilage lesions (in 70% of the cases), ligamentous injuries (60%, mostly ruptures of the calcaneofibular ligament), and anterior dislocations of the peroneal tendons (30%) caused by a pure ligamentous or osseous avulsion of the tendon sheath at the distal fibula. Depending on the extent and characteristic of these concomitant injuries, an operative repair might be indicated at the time of fracture repair.

DIAGNOSIS

LTPF has often been misdiagnosed as a lateral ankle sprain, especially in snowboarder injuries.[6] The diagnosis can usually be made by means of a detailed history, clinical examination, and use of standard plain radiographs. Typically, there is a localized tender spot 1 cm inferior and anterior to the tip of the distal fibula.[13] The fracture can be visualized on 1 (or both) of the 2 plain radiographs. In the lateral view, an intact lateral talar process (LTP) has a typical symmetric V-shaped contour. In cases of a displaced fracture, this symmetry often is lost and the LTP is projected in a crooked or

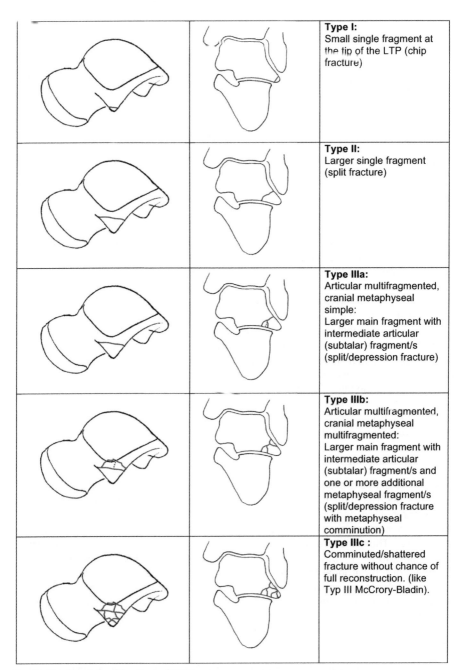

		Type I: Small single fragment at the tip of the LTP (chip fracture)
		Type II: Larger single fragment (split fracture)
		Type IIIa: Articular multifragmented, cranial metaphyseal simple: Larger main fragment with intermediate articular (subtalar) fragment/s (split/depression fracture)
		Type IIIb: Articular multifragmented, cranial metaphyseal multifragmented: Larger main fragment with intermediate articular (subtalar) fragment/s and one or more additional metaphyseal fragment/s (split/depression fracture with metaphyseal comminution)
		Type IIIc : Comminuted/shattered fracture without chance of full reconstruction. (like Typ III McCrory-Bladin).

Fig. 2. Modified classification of LTPF.

otherwise asymmetric V-shape (**Fig. 3**). This appearance is designated as a positive V-sign.[13,14] The authors recommend further imaging with a CT scan for all cases of diagnosed fracture as well as cases of suspected fracture. Only a CT with standard 2-D reconstructions (sagittal and frontal) allows proper assessment of the fracture

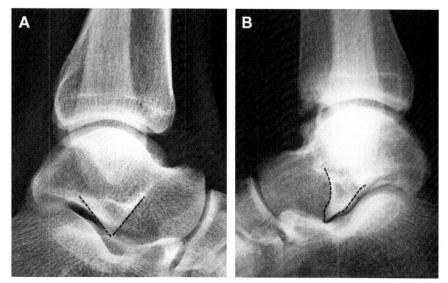

Fig. 3. (A) Normal V-sign on contralateral noninjured side. (B) Pathologic V-sign on injured side.

morphology and degree of displacement.[15] 3-D reconstructions are helpful to assess the extent of the metaphyseal comminution, which might be important for the reduction maneuver (cortical reads) and the choice of implant for fracture stabilization. Alternatively, the MRI allows visualization of associated soft-tissue and cartilaginous injuries, but is less useful to analyze the bony trauma.

THERAPY

The treatment of LTPF is chosen according to the type and displacement of the fracture (**Fig. 4**).

In general, nondisplaced (or only minimally displaced) fractures of any type can be addressed conservatively using an immobilization in a splint or a cast for at least 6 weeks. During that time only partial weight bearing (10 kg) is allowed. The same type treatment is advised for most type I fractures independent of the grade of displacement. In cases of indicated surgery for another reason (eg, peroneal tendon dislocation), the small single type I fragment can be addressed either by removal or—if large enough—by single screw fixation.

Because most of the type II and type III fractures are found displaced, surgery is necessary.

In type II and many type IIIa fractures a screw fixation (2 mm × 1.5–2.4 mm) is sufficient. In cases of anatomic reduction, there is a large bony contact area created between the main fragment and the (cranially) intact talus (load sharing situation) and, therefore, the implants do not become strongly stressed.

In type IIIb fractures, however, due to the (cranial) metaphyseal comminution, no load-sharing can be achieved. Therefore, the authors advise using a small T-plate for fixation in a buttress function.

Another advantage of the surgical treatment is the functional postoperative recovery protocol, which in most cases can be began right after surgery. The impairment of articular and muscular functions is much less compared with the conservative treatment (rigid fixation in a cast). Therefore, surgery frequently is preferred by young athletes, due to the earlier return to regular sport activities.

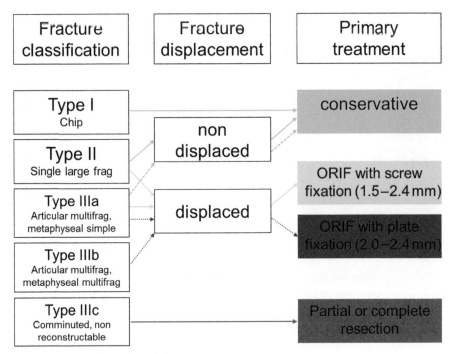

Fig. 4. Treatment algorithm of the LTPF.

SURGICAL TECHNIQUE
Timing

A displaced LTPF can be fixed a few days (3–7) after initial trauma when the soft tissue swelling has regressed. Immediate surgery is possible in cases of isolated fractures with minimal swelling (first 6 hours). Timing is highly depending on associated injuries of the foot and ankle, as, for example, in polytrauma cases.

Position of the Patient

Positioning depends on potentially present associated injuries. In isolated fracture, as in most cases, a lateral position is preferred. Alternatively, the patient can be placed supine on the operating table with a large pad under the ipsilateral buttock to rotate the leg internally. This turns the hindfoot in a more lateral position. The authors routinely use a thigh tourniquet, which is inflated after elevating the leg for partial exsanguination.[16]

Anesthesia

As in most cases of lower extremity surgery, a general or spinal anesthesia can be performed. A perioperative antibiotic prophylaxis (eg, cefazolin, 2 g or 3 g) reduces the perioperative risk of infection.[17,18]

Landmarks

The landmarks of lateral hindfoot include the distal fibula, calcaneal tuberosity with the lateral wall of the calcaneus, tuberosity of the base of fifth metatarsal bone (MT V), and the anterior process of the calcaneus. The tip of the LTP is located typically 1 cm inferior and anterior to the distal tip of the fibula.

Approach

Two possible approaches are available. The Ollier approach has been described as a transverse access at the level of the subtalar joint.[19,20] This approach allows an optimal access to the LTP and the subtalar joint but is less helpful when the posterior part of the distal fibula should be reached or a ruptured peroneal tendon sheath repair is required. Its oblique course runs over the sural and/or superficial peroneal nerve and may endanger it.

The authors prefer a slightly curved skin incision starting at the posterior and inferior end of the fibula, running straight over the anterior process of the calcaneus until ending above the upper border of the base of MT V (**Fig. 5**). The course of the incision runs dorsally and parallel to the sural nerve. Therefore, the risk of neuropraxia is reduced.

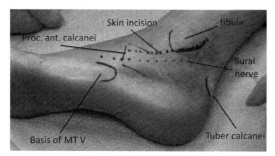

Fig. 5. Landmarks at lateral hindfoot. proc.ant. calcanei, anterior process of calcaneus.

The subcutaneous layer and superficial fascia are divided (Scarpa) and the peroneal tendon sheath opened to expose the peroneal tendons. This is an important step to address any potential injury of the tendon sheath leading to anterior tendon dislocation and for repair of the peroneal tendon as well. As a next step, the anterior talofibular ligament (ATFL) is exposed, which in most cases is intact.[13] Below the ATFL, the tip of the LTP is now easily palpable. The talofibular and subtalar joint capsules are incised (if not yet ruptured by the injury). In cases of anterocranial fracture extension, it might be necessary to either divide or (better) osteotomize the attachment of the ATFL. Then, the fracture is assessed by rotating the main fracture fragment anteriorly and cranially combined with manual eversion of the hindfoot, which provides access to the subtalar joint. In cases of complex fractures (especially type IIIb fracture), the authors advise to use a small distractor, which can be anchored between the distal tibia, distal fibula, or talar neck cranially and the calcaneus caudally (**Fig. 6**). After evacuation of the hemarthrosis, small chondral and/or osteochondral debris are usually found and washed out of the joint (see **Fig. 23**A).

Reduction

The rotation of the main fragment allows access to existing (or potentially existing) intermediate talar articular fragments of the subtalar joint (all type III fractures). When the fracture gaps are cleaned from clotted hematomas and other debris, the reduction starts with the most medially located intermediate fragment. For this reduction step, it is important to align the calcaneus correctly to the talus by releasing the everted position of the hindfoot. Usually this intermediate fragment

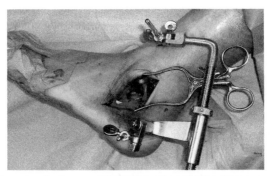

Fig. 6. Use of a distractor for better visibility into the subtalar joint.

cannot be (temporarily) fixed but usually stays in place after reduction. The next step is to reduce the main fragment by pushing it medially onto the intact talus (or the already reduced intermediate fragment) and caudally toward the subtalar articular facet of the calcaneus. It is then fixed temporarily with 1 or 2 small Kirschner (K)-wires. In cases of metaphyseal (cranial) comminution, these fragments, if still attached to soft tissues (periosteum, capsule), can be placed in the fracture gap aiming for anatomic reduction even of this extra-articular part. If large enough, they can be further fixed by small K-wires (**Fig. 7**).

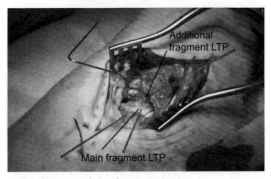

Fig. 7. Temporary K-wire fixation of the fragments.

Fixation

Implant selection depends on the fracture type (see **Fig. 2**). In cases of type I and type II, a screw fixation (lag screw technique) alone with 2 screws (or 1 screw and 1 small antirotational K-wire in small fragments) is sufficient (see **Figs. 11–13**). Even in type IIIa (when the main fragment is large and the intermediate fragments small), screw fixation might be sufficient. In more complex fractures (type IIIb), the authors advise using a small T-plate (1.5–2.4 mm) in buttress function (see **Fig. 23**B; Figs. **15–24**). The cranial T-bar of this plate is usually placed onto the base of the talar neck just anterior of the cartilage, which faces the distal fibula (**Fig. 8**). Before definitive plate fixation, an impingement of the fibula by the plate has to be ruled out by maximal extension (dorsiflexion) of the upper ankle joint. The authors never use a bone graft, but in cases of metaphyseal comminution (type IIIb fracture), small fracture debris has been used to fill the metaphyseal defect.

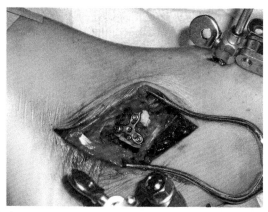

Fig. 8. T-plate with the superior T-bar placed just anterior to the talar cartilage facing the fibula and the caudal part 1 mm to 2 mm above the distal end of the LTP not interfering with the posterior facet of the calcaneus (not visible on this figure, because the joint is still under distraction).

Intraoperative Radiographic Assessment

An intraoperative fluoroscopic control is performed using the classic ankle projections in lateral and anteroposterior view, completed with Broden view to visualize the subtalar joint. The original Broden view is done in an internal rotation position of the foot of 30° to 45° and an inclination of 10° to 40° depending on the part of the subtalar facet of the calcaneus addressed. Articular steps and gaps are usually visualized well when they are located in a fracture plane parallel to the x-ray beam. This is the case when using the Broden view for intra-articular calcaneal fractures, but it is not true for LTPFs, where the main fracture plane is approximately 90° rotated compared with the fracture plane on the posterior facet of calcaneal fractures. Therefore, in the authors' experience, a reversed Broden view in external rotation of the foot of approximately 45° to 60° and 10° to 20° inclination allows for the best assessment of reduction quality of the articular facet of the LTP[13] (see **Figs. 11**A, **15**C, and **18**D).

Associated Injuries

If present, further injuries are addressed at the same operation. This includes screw fixation of further fractures (talar neck or anterior process of the talus) and repair of avulsed or torn ligaments (ATFL rare). The calcaneotalar ligament is usually avulsed distally. Quite a time ago, the authors used to refix it there, but in recent years this

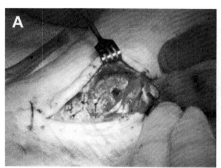
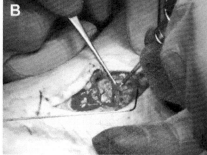

Fig. 9. (A, B) Refixation of osseous avulsion of the peroneal tendon sheath with a 2.0-mm screw.

manouver has been stopped due to the risk of sural nerve damage and because it did not seem to be essential because it never ended up in ankle instability.

In cases of peroneal tendon dislocation, refixation of the avulsed tendon sheath can be accomplished at the distal fibular level by means of transosseous sutures or alternatively using 1 or 2 small bone anchors. In cases of osseous avulsion, a fixation with 1 or 2 small screws or a bone stapler can be performed (**Fig. 9**; see **Figs. 19** and **20**).

POSTOPERATIVE CARE

Generally speaking, after a short bed rest (1 day to 2 days), the patient commences a mobilization on crutches and partial weight bearing (10 kg–15 kg) for a duration of 6 weeks.

Perfect patient compliance may allow a functional postoperative protocol without immobilization. If ligament or tendon sheath repair has been performed, however, this cannot be done. In such cases, the ankle should be protected for 6 weeks in a walking boot. After 6 weeks, loading is rapidly increased so that after 8 weeks full weight bearing is allowed. Higher loading activities (jumping, snowboarding, climbing, ball games, and so forth) are recommended 3 months to 4 months after initial trauma.

Clinical and radiographic follow-up is performed 6 weeks, 12 weeks, and 1 year after surgery.

Implant removal is not necessary but can be considered in cases of irritation. In cases of plate fixation, the authors are usually inclined to plan a removal.

Prognosis

As in most articular injuries, the outcome depends on 2 factors: (1) the degree of traumatic cartilage damage and (2) the accuracy of the restoration of joint surface congruity. A nondisplaced fracture might have only minimal cartilage damage and, therefore, usually leads to an excellent result after conservative treatment. Comminuted and quite displaced fractures often result after a high-energy mechanism and have a higher degree of cartilage damage and, therefore, less favorable outcome. This is also the case even if treated optimally.

The outcome after LTPF is generally favorable. An early recognition of the injury and proper treatment regime provides a good base for an adequate outcome. A larger series of conservatively (nondisplaced fractures) and operatively (displaced fractures) treated LTPFs was able to demonstrate good clinical results, with a mean American Orthopedic Foot and Ankle Society hindfoot score of 94 points (maximum 100).[13] Similar excellent results have been reported by other investigators.[2,8] These series represent, however, results of a special injury mechanism (snowboarding), which might be more favorable compared with other injuries, such as car accidents or falls from heights or climbing. Radiographically, 50% of the cases showed a mild to moderate osteoarthritis at the subtalar joint, mainly in cases of displaced fracture and higher degree of cartilage damage and operative treatment.[13]

Complications

The first complication occurs when missing or misinterpreting the fracture as an ankle sprain.[15,21] In this case, a malunion or nonunion may result causing a chronic pain syndrome requiring late surgical treatment. The options vary from late fixation to corrective osteotomy or complete resection. The same complications can occur after conservative treatment,[22] especially when the initial displacement of the fracture was underestimated, for example, when relying on conventional radiographs only.

Surgical treatment is mostly successful concerning fracture union in correct position. The approach is safe and wound healing problems are rare and not mentioned in literature. They remain possible, however, when considering improper timing of surgery and/or neglected risk factors of the patient. Nonetheless, it is important to avoid damaging of the thin skin by means of inadequate usage of hooks or retractors. The approach may endanger the lateral dorsal cutaneous nerve (end branch of the sural nerve), which runs caudal and parallel to the approach discussed previously but crosses the standard subtalar approach (Ollier).

Osteoarthritis often occurs even after correct treatment. This is not considered a complication, unless the fracture is not adequately treated, as described previously. Most of the displaced LTPFs are accompanied by minor or major cartilage damage of the subtalar joint, leading to some degree of osteoarthritis . Besides conservative treatment with physical therapy, analgesics, and intraarticular injections, operative procedures, such as open or arthroscopic débridement, or, finally, a subtalar fusion, might be necessary in certain cases. Fortunately, this is rarely needed (in the authors' experience <5%), although long-term results (>5 years) have not been published.[20,23]

In cases of implant irritation, removal is recommended 4 months to 6 months after initial surgery at the earliest (see **Figs. 25** and **26**).

CASE EXAMPLES
Case 1: Lateral Talar Process Fracture Type II

A 21-year-old man suffered an ankle sprain during landing after performing a backflip from a fountain. Conventional radiographs show some horizontal nondisplaced

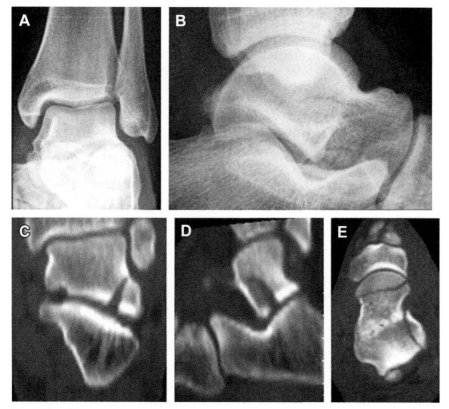

Fig. 10. (*A, B*) Preoperative radiograph, anteroposterior/lateral. (*C–E*) Preoperative CT scan.

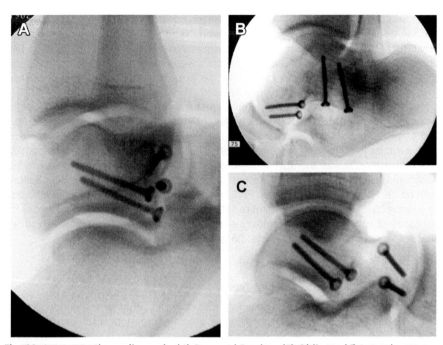

Fig. 11. Intraoperative radiograph. (*A*) Reversed Broden. (*B*) Oblique. (*C*) Lateral.

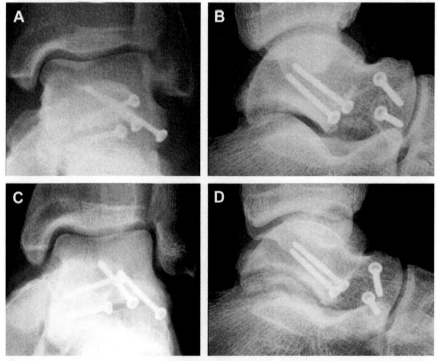

Fig. 12. (*A, B*) Postoperative radiograph, anteroposterior/lateral. (*C, D*). One-year follow-up radiograph.

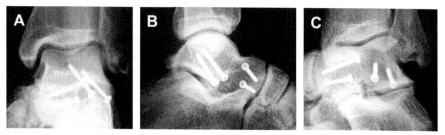

Fig. 13. Three-year follow-up radiograph. (*A*) Anteroposterior. (*B*) Lateral. (*C*) Broden view.

fracture lines in the talar neck (**Fig. 10**A, B). The CT scan reveals not only the displaced type II fracture of the lateral process but also a collateral injury with a nondisplaced transverse fracture of the anterior process of the talus (**Fig. 10**C–E). Both fracture components were treated with ORIF (lag screw fixation) using 1 anterolateral approach, as described previously. Intraoperative fluoroscopy in different projections demonstrates anatomic reduction (**Fig. 11**A–C). After 3 years and a normal recovery, the very active patient desired implant removal due to some pain after running and some meteosensitivity. On radiograph, only minimal degenerative changes were detected (**Figs. 12** and **13**).

Case 2: Lateral Talar Process Fracture Type IIIa

A 28-year-old man sustained an ankle sprain after a climbing fall. He presented with swelling, pain, and inability to load his injured foot. Initially in the emergency

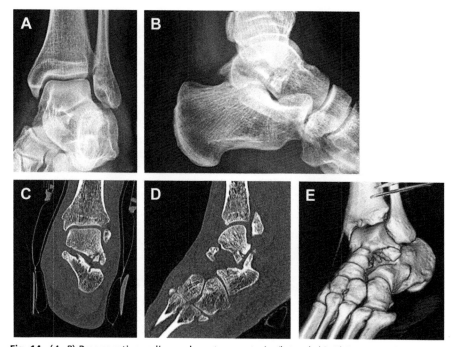

Fig. 14. (*A, B*) Preoperative radiograph, anteroposterior/lateral. (*C, D*) Preoperative CT scan. (*E*) Preoperative CT scan 3-D reco.

room, the fracture was missed, although it was clearly visible on the conventional radiographs with a positive V-sign (**Fig. 14**A, B). Some days later, the correct diagnosis was made and confirmed by a CT scan (**Fig. 14**C–E), whereby a nondisplaced talar neck fracture as a typical collateral injury was detected. The displaced fracture can be classified as type IIIa (intra-articular multifragmented but metaphyseal simple without additional fragments). It was treated with ORIF using a small T-plate due to the several intraarticular fragments making an isolated screw fixation precarious. The talar neck was secured by 1 anteroposterior lag screw. Intraoperatively, a larger osteochondral flake fracture of the posterior facet of the calcaneus was found and fixed using resorbable pins (**Fig. 15**). The postoperative mobilization was with an aircast and partial weight bearing for 6 weeks, with increase to full weight bearing 10 weeks postoperatively. After 17 months, the implants were removed because of some residual pain when performing high-impact sports, such as hiking and rock climbing (**Fig. 16**).

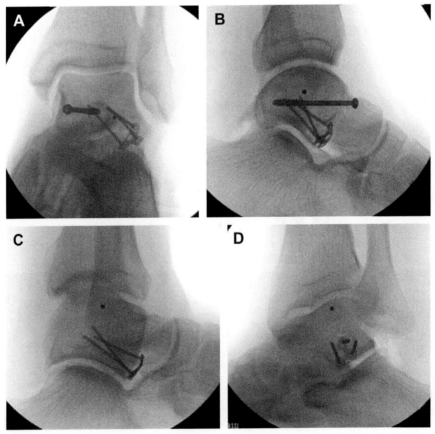

Fig. 15. (*A, B*) Intraoperative radiograph, anteroposterior/lateral. (*C, D*) Intraoperative radiograph, reversed Broden and Broden.

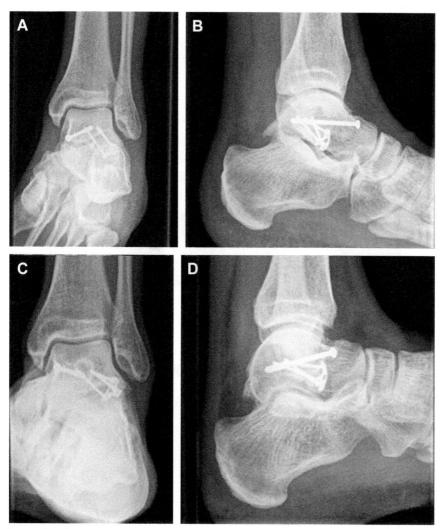

Fig. 16. (*A, B*) Postoperative radiograph, anteroposterior/lateral. (*C, D*) One-year follow-up radiograph anteroposterior/lateral.

Case 3: Lateral Talar Process Fracture Type IIIb

A 34-year-old man sprained his left ankle during work on a building yard (Video 1). He presented with pain, swelling, and inability to bear weight. The imaging demonstrates a type IIIb fracture of the LTP and the indirect sign of having had a peroneal tendon dislocation as a typical collateral injury: on conventional radiograph (**Fig. 17**A), as on CT scan (**Fig. 17**E), the osseous avulsed tendon sheath is clearly visible. The fracture was fixed with a small T-plate and an additional lag screw for a larger separate metaphyseal fragment as well as a single 2.0mm screw for the fixation of the bony fragment of the peroneal tendon sheath (**Figs. 18** and **19**). After 15 weeks, the patient was pain free under full weight bearing. Five months after injury the patient restarted work as a constructor (**Fig. 20**).

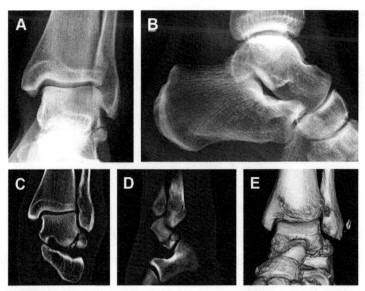

Fig. 17. (*A, B*) Preoperative radiograph, anteroposterior/lateral. (*C, D*) Preoperative CT scan. (*E*) Preoperative CT scan, 3-D reco.

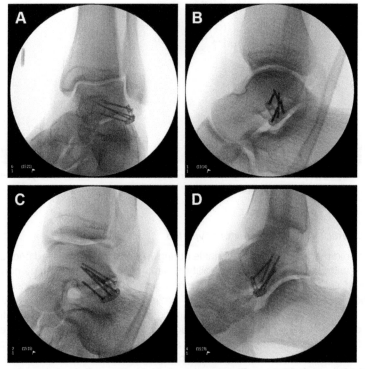

Fig. 18. Intraoperative radiograph. (*A, B*) Anteroposterior/lateral. (*C*) Broden, (*D*) Reversed Broden.

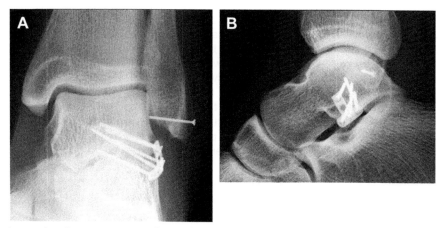

Fig. 19. (*A*, *B*) Postoperative radiograph, anteroposterior/lateral.

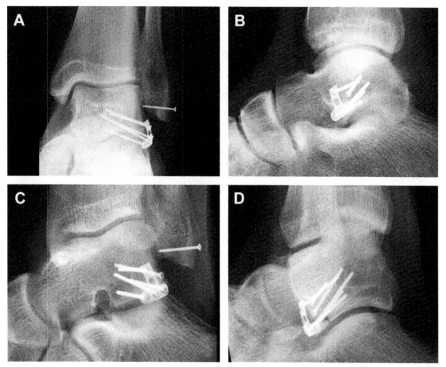

Fig. 20. Three-month follow-up radiograph. (*A*, *B*) Anteroposterior/lateral. (*C*) Broden. (*D*) Reversed Broden.

Case 4: Lateral Talar Process Fracture Type IIIb (Type IIIc)

A 43-year-old man with a climbing fall sustained a comminuted fracture (**Fig. 21** A–E). This could be classified as type IIIc, but intraoperatively the authors realized that a reconstruction was feasible so it was downgraded to a type IIIb fracture (see **Fig. 4**). The initial swelling was massive so that operative treatment was performed 10 days after trauma (**Fig. 22**). Many small osteochondral fragments, avulsed from the posterolateral border of the calcaneal facet, had to be removed (see **Fig. 23**A) and the comminuted fracture was fixed with a small T-plate in buttress function. Because of increased pain in the subtalar joint and possible implant irritation (which was placed very close to the posterior facet [see

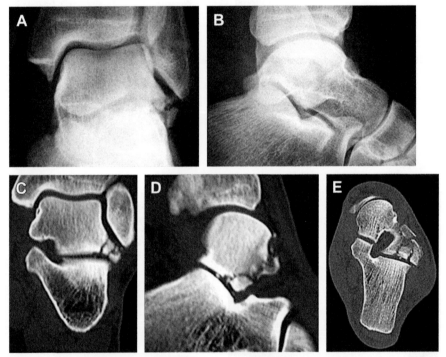

Fig. 21. (A, B). Preoperative radiograph, anteroposterior/lateral. (C–E) Preoperative CT scan, anteroposterior/lateral and axial views.

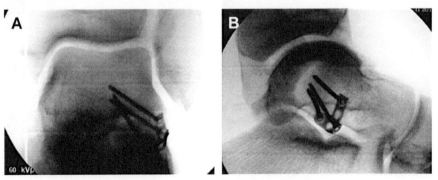

Fig. 22. (A, B) Intraoperative radiograph, anteroposterior/lateral.

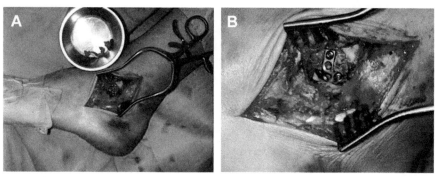

Fig. 23. (A) Perioperative pictures showing the removed osteochondral small debris (in metallic cup). (B) T-plate placed in front of the cartilage facing the fibula and rather close to the cartilage of the posterior facet of the calcaneus.

Fig. 23B and 24]), it was removed 6 months after fracture fixation. The follow-up CT scan (Fig. 25) shows a marked osteoarthritis of the subtalar joint (joint space narrowing and central osteolysis/defect) and the patient suffered a chronic regional pain syndrome. A neurostimulator implantation followed, which was used for 2 years until complete symptom regression. The 4-year follow-up radiographs demonstrate a stable nonincreasing osteoarthritis (Fig. 26). Ten years after the injury, the patient has only minimal residual pain and is not in need of any special treatment.

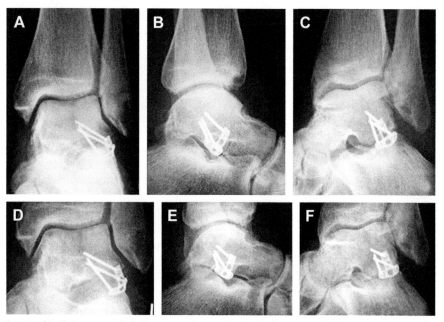

Fig. 24. (A–C) Seven-week follow-up radiograph. (D–F) Three-month follow-up radiograph.

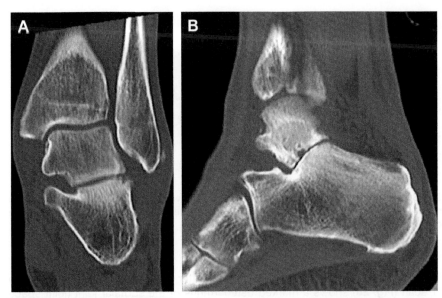

Fig. 25. (*A, B*) CT scan 8 months after implant removal.

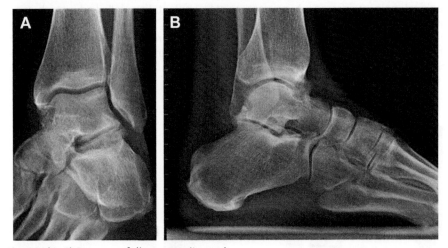

Fig. 26. (*A, B*) Four-year follow-up radiograph.

ACKNOWLEDGMENTS

The authors would like to thank Dr M. Spasojević for his accurate proofreading and English language correction.

SUPPLEMENTARY DATA

Supplementary data related to this article can be found online at https://doi.org/10.1016/j.fcl.2018.04.009.

REFERENCES

1. Summers JN, Murdoch MM. Fractures of the talus: a comprehensive review. Clin Podiatr Med Surg 2012;29(2):188–203.

2. Valderrabano V, Perren T, Ryf C, et al. Snowboarder's talus fracture. Am J Sports Med 2005;33(6):871–80.
3. Chan GM, Yoshida D. Fracture of the lateral process of the talus associated with snowboarding. Ann Emerg Med 2003;41(6):854–8.
4. Miller S. Fractures of the lateral process of the talus. Foot 1996;6(4):188–92.
5. Kramer IF, Brouwers L, Brink PRG, et al. Snowboarders' ankle. BMJ Case Rep 2014. https://doi.org/10.1136/bcr-2014-204220.
6. Kirkpatrick DP, Hunter RE, Janes PC, et al. The snowboarder's foot and ankle. Am J Sports Med 1998;26(2):271–7.
7. Berkowitz MJ, Kim DH. Process and tubercle fractures of the hindfoot. J Am Acad Orthop Surg 2005;13(8):492–502.
8. Perera A, Baker JF, Lui DF, et al. The management and outcome of lateral process fracture of the talus. Foot Ankle Surg 2010;16(1):15–20.
9. Mukherjee SK, Pringle RM, Baxter AB. Fracture of the lateral talar process. J Bone Jt Surg 1974;56b(12):340–2. Available at: http://www.ncbi.nlm.nih.gov/pubmed/1480256.
10. Hawkins LG. Fracture of the lateral process of the talus. J Bone Joint Surg Am 1965;47:1170–5.
11. Boon AJ, Smith J, Zobitz ME, et al. Snowboarder's talus fracture mechanism of injury. Am J Sports Med 2001;29(3):333–8.
12. McCrory P, Bladin C. Fractures of the lateral process of the talus: a clinical review. Clin J Sport Med 1996;6:124–8.
13. von Knoch F, Reckord U, von Knoch M, et al. Fracture of the lateral process of the talus in snowboarders. J Bone Joint Surg Br 2007;89(6):772–7.
14. Jentzsch T, Hasler A, Renner N, et al. The V sign in lateral talar process fractures: an experimental study using a foot and ankle model. BMC Musculoskelet Disord 2017;18(1):284.
15. Noble J, Royle SG. Fracture of the lateral process of the talus: computed tomographic scan diagnosis. Br J Sports Med 1992;26(4):245–6.
16. Noordin S, McEwen JA, Kragh CJF, et al. Surgical tourniquets in orthopaedics. J Bone Joint Surg Am 2009;91(12):2958–67.
17. Yamada K, Matsumoto K, Tokimura F, et al. Are bone and serum cefazolin concentrations adequate for antimicrobial prophylaxis? Clin Orthop Relat Res 2011;469(12):3486–94.
18. Fletcher N. Prevention of perioperative infection. J Bone Jt Surg 2007;89(7):1605.
19. Schepers T. The sinus tarsi approach in displaced intra-articular calcaneal fractures: a systematic review. Int Orthop 2011;35(5):697–703.
20. Schepers T, Kieboom BCT, Bessems GHJM, et al. Subtalar versus triple arthrodesis after intra-articular calcaneal fractures. Strategies Trauma Limb Reconstr 2010;5(2):97–103.
21. Young KW, Park YU, Kim JS, et al. Misdiagnosis of talar body or neck fractures as ankle sprains in low energy traumas. Clin Orthop Surg 2016;8(3):303–9.
22. Parsons SJ. Relation between the occurrence of bony union and outcome for fractures of the lateral process of the talus: a case report and analysis of published reports. Br J Sports Med 2003;37(3):274–6.
23. Ohl X, Harisboure A, Hemery X, et al. Long-term follow-up after surgical treatment of talar fractures: twenty cases with an average follow-up of 7.5 years. Int Orthop 2011;35(1):93–9.

Update on Subtalar Joint Instability

Thomas Mittlmeier, MD, PhD[a],*, Stefan Rammelt, MD, PhD[b]

KEYWORDS

- Subtalar joint • Subtalar instability • Interosseous talocalcaneal ligament
- Lateral ankle ligament complex • Medial subtalar instability • Diagnostic algorithm
- Ligamentous reconstruction

KEY POINTS

- Subtalar joint stability is ensured by both the osseous geometry of the talocalcaneal joint and the ligaments at the medial and lateral aspect of the ankle joint, the sinus and canalis tarsi, and the talocalcaneonavicular joint.
- Subtalar joint function, the three-dimensional interaction of the ankle and subtalar joint complex, which can mutually compensate for functional deficits, are still poorly understood.
- Subtalar joint instability is a more frequent phenomenon than is generally assumed. Subtalar instability refers to lateral and medial subtalar joint instability.
- The clinical diagnosis should rely on several parameters being part of a diagnostic algorithm.
- The therapeutic portfolio comprises nonsurgical and surgical treatment in which anatomic reconstruction should be given preference rather than nonanatomic methods, per the inherent risk portfolio.

INTRODUCTION

Within the broad topic of lateral ankle instability the involvement of the subtalar joint is frequently neglected despite about 25% of the cases presenting with combined injuries of the lateral ankle and the subtalar joint.[1–7] In particular, the calcaneofibular ligament (CFL) bridges the subtalar joint and contributes essentially to subtalar joint stability in case of injury.[6] Therefore, the assumption that subtalar ligamentous injuries represent a rare entity is not correct.[3–5] Both isolated lesions of the CFL and the

Disclosure: The authors have nothing to disclose.
[a] Department of Trauma, Hand and Reconstructive Surgery, Rostock University Medical Center, Schillingallee 35, Rostock D-18057, Germany; [b] University Center for Orthopedics and Traumatology, University Hospital "Carl Gustav Carus", TU Dresden, Fetscherstr. 74, Dresden D-01307, Germany
* Corresponding author.
E-mail address: Thomas.mittlmeier@med.uni-rostock.de

interosseous talocalcaneal ligament (ITCL) are observed in less than 1%, which suggests a typical manifestation of combined ligamentous injuries; for example, of the CFL, anterior fibulotalar ligament (AFTL), and components of the subtalar ligaments, eventually leading to a multi-dimensional instability.[3,4,8] Because of similar injury mechanisms and clinical symptoms, subtalar joint instability (STI) is often missed or misinterpreted.[3,4] Taking into account that around 20% of the patients who sustain an acute ankle sprain will develop chronic ankle instability (CAI), a comparable number of patients might present with chronic STI as well.[3,4,9] Even repetitive microtrauma of the interosseous and neighboring ligaments may contribute to a chronic ligamentous elongation and consecutive STI.[3,4] Furthermore, STI does not simply comprise a further subtype of lateral ankle joint instability, because relevant structures of the subtalar joint ligaments such as the ITCL and the tibiocalcaneal fascicle of the deltoid ligament represent restraints against pronation forces. Thus, the concept of peritalar stability, as referred to by Hintermann and colleagues,[10] allows for a more comprehensive view of the variants of STI.[10,11]

In the past, nonanatomic tenodesis techniques using a part of the peroneus longus or brevis tendon or an allograft were popular in the treatment of CAI. Their clinical success, at least a part of it, might have been caused by the recognition that a concomitant STI has been addressed as well.[3,4,12] A recent publication to define a consensus about the clinical approach in patients with chronic lateral ankle instability revealed that there was a consensus about neither the diagnostic nor the therapeutic algorithm in STI among the wide and international spectrum of experts involved.[13] If the major publications on STI during the last 10 years are analyzed, it seems that some of the dissent within the recommendations are even caused by different definitions of the anatomic structures and interpretation of their biomechanical relevance.[4,9,14] Most publications on the topic are cumulative case series with limited numbers of subjects included. Therefore, the topic of STI and its clinical management is still far from being evidence based. In the following, a clinically oriented approach to ligamentous STI is attempted, including the recently published literature, which has not been included in other reviews on the topic[5,7] and points to contradictory statements. Subtalar joint dislocations or concomitant fractures or fracture-dislocations are not discussed because they represent an entity of their own and hardly ever lead to chronic STI.[3,4,11] (These injuries are addressed in Rammelt and colleagues' article, Traumatic Injury to the Subtalar Joint, in this issue.)

SUBTALAR JOINT ANATOMY AND BIOMECHANICS

The complex geometry of the articulating bones and the corresponding ligaments both essentially contribute to subtalar joint stability. The functional unit of the talocalcaneonavicular (TCN) joint (the coxa pedis) and the subtalar joint provides a different amount of stability because of the geometric correspondence of the joint surfaces and guides mobility and motion.[14–17] Inversion and eversion, which are generally attributed to subtalar joint function, occur simultaneously at the TCN and subtalar joints.[14] Meanwhile, a single oblique axis of motion at the subtalar joint level, as was assumed in earlier studies, has been rejected in favor of a bundle of instantaneous axes because of the irregular shape of the subtalar joint facets.[3,4] From a clinical viewpoint the assumption of a uniaxial motion of the subtalar joint where the calcaneus with respect to the talus rotates from dorsolateral to medioplantar and the coincidence of this axis with the plane of motion of hindfoot inversion/eversion might still seem to be an acceptable and simplified working concept.[11] However, eversion is intrinsically linked with extension (dorsiflexion), pronation, and adduction, whereas inversion is linked with flexion, supination, and adduction of the foot.[4] In eversion, maximum contact caused by joint surface congruency at the posterior subtalar joint generates a high degree of inherent stability.[14] Otherwise, the ligaments contribute to subtalar joint stability. There has been some confusion about the nomenclature of the relevant ligaments of the subtalar joint in anatomic and biomechanical studies as well.[18] A topographic assignment seems to be more appropriate than a general and dichotomous distinction of intrinsic and extrinsic structures.[12,14] Within the sinus and canalis tarsi the following ligamentous structures can be separated from medial to lateral: the ITCL; the medial root of the inferior extensor retinaculum (IER); the anterior talocalcaneal ligament (ATCL), which reinforces the anterior subtalar joint capsule and has traditionally been considered to represent a part of the ITCL despite the regular presence of adipose tissue between these two structures; the oblique talocalcaneal ligament (OTCL), which has been termed the cervical ligament; and the intermediate and lateral roots of the IER. The roots of the IER insert immediately behind the footprint of the cervical ligament and the lateral calcaneal wall, and the medial root of the IER crosses medially and partially blends with the fibers of the ITCL[14] (**Fig. 1**). A recent cadaveric dissection study focused on the geometry of the OTCL, and a trapezoidal geometry of the ligament with an average width of 9.15 mm superiorly and 11.9 mm inferiorly and a mean thickness of 0.62 mm at the anterior-superior edge and 1.2 mm at the posterior-inferior edge was verified.[19] On the lateral aspect of the subtalar joint, the CFL is the only component of the lateral collateral ligaments that crosses both the ankle and subtalar joint. Thus, the CFL works against anterolateral rotational instability in conjunction with the inconstant and weak lateral talocalcaneal ligament (LTCL), which runs from the lateral talar process to its insertion on the lateral calcaneal wall just medial to the CFL[14] (see **Fig. 1**). On the medial aspect, the anterior tibiosubtalar part of the deltoid ligament, which

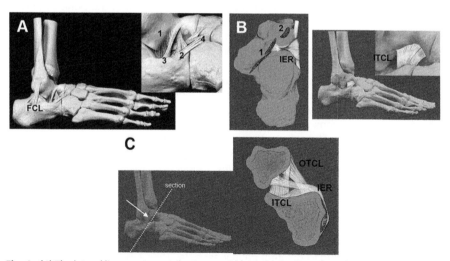

Fig. 1. (*A*) The lateral ligaments contributing to ankle and subtalar joint stability. Fibulocalcaneal ligament (FCL): 1, ITCL; 2, OTCL (cervical ligament); 3, ATCL; 4, bifurcate ligament. (*B*) Left: insertion points of the 3 components of the IER. 1, medial and intermediate; 2, lateral. Right: removing the IER, the ATCL, and the cervical ligament opens the view to the bilaminar V-shaped bundle of the ITCL. (*C*) The view to the talocalcaneal joint from behind shows how the IER blends with the ITCL and the OTCL. The arrow in (*C*) points to the sinus tarsi. (*From* Mittlmeier T, Wichelhaus A. Subtalar joint instability. Eur J Trauma Emerg Surg 2015;41:624; with permission.)

is in close relation to the superomedial part of the spring ligament, contributes to subtalar joint stability in sliding, rolling, and torsion.[14,20] Hintermann and colleagues[10,20,21] formulated the observational model of peritalar instability, in which the ITCL ligament and the ligaments of the talonavicular joint play a fundamental role in the development of chronic instability. The model is helpful for the description of the interaction between the ankle and the subtalar joint; for example, in compensating for horizontal plane deformity and instability at the ankle joint level through the subtalar joint despite these mechanisms of interaction still being poorly understood.[10,21]

There have been various cadaver studies published to further describe the mechanical contribution of the individual ligaments described earlier to subtalar joint stability, with conflicting results. Although there have been several reports about the paramount role of the CFL for ankle and subtalar joint stability, questioning the relevance of the ITCL and its neighboring structures[3,4,6,22] (**Fig. 2**), others have pointed to the equivalent importance of the ligamentous components of the sinus and canalis tarsi.[11,18,23,24] The Y-shaped ITCL can be compared with the cruciate ligaments of the knee with respect to its stabilizing function at the subtalar joint and the presence of proprioceptive nerve endings within the ligament.[25,26] Although the mechanical constraints under three-dimensional (3D) loading conditions can mimic the physiologic conditions, the missing muscular activation represents a major drawback with cadaveric testing.

This problem might be solved by in vivo assessment of subtalar joint function. With the help of computed tomography (CT) scanning, the range of subtalar joint motion has been measured in vivo with a range of motion from 5° to 16° (mean, 11°) to 37° ± 5°,[27] which is substantially lower than the clinical evaluation in which goniometer measurements resulted in a range of subtalar joint motion from 39° to 54°, pointing to the role of the soft tissues and concomitant talocrural motion.[28] Recently, gait analysis using high-speed dual fluoroscopy and 3D modeling of the bone segments via CT scans in a limited series of patients with CAI revealed that, during balanced heel testing, patients with CAI displayed more tibiotalar and subtalar kinematic variation compared with control subjects.[29] Surprisingly, during treadmill walking at low gait velocity, less overall joint translation has been registered in patients with CAI compared with healthy controls.[29] These results indirectly confirm previous cadaver studies in which the assessment of anatomic landmarks seemed to be superior to that of bone markers.[18] Moreover, 3D analysis using dynamic CT scans in healthy and cadaver specimens with sequential sectioning of ligaments contributing to subtalar joint stability,[30] dynamic stress MRI,[31] or quantitative MRI with 3D reconstruction[32] might offer noninvasive tools for assessment of the biomechanical consequences of STI. A clinically relevant in vitro model of medial STI has not yet been established.

CLASSIFICATION OF SUBTALAR JOINT INSTABILITY

Usuelli and colleagues[8] provided a comprehensive approach to categorizing CAI and STI in which they included different causal aspects. Their type 1 represents isolated axial deviation at the ankle or subtalar joint and combined multilevel deformities that typically manifest in patients with congenital or acquired deformities; for example, following secondary arthritic changes. Type 2 refers to ligamentous instabilities in which a combined CAI and STI is considered separately from a mere manifestation at the subtalar joint level, and type 3 includes any form of functional instability. Kato[33] indicated that a shallower angle of the subtalar joint facet or hereditary motor

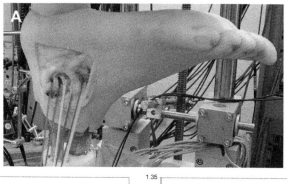

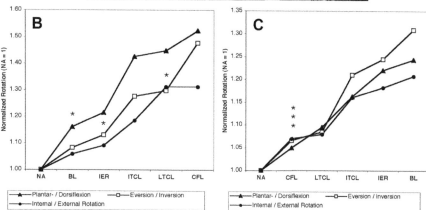

Fig. 2. (*A*) Cadaver specimens mounted upside down within the cardanic ankle joint simulator with 4 components of the lateral ligaments bridging the subtalar joint marked with vessel loops: yellow, bifurcate ligament; red, IER; white, LTCL; blue, CFL. The ITCL is below the IER and is not visible here. (*B*) Increasing subtalar instability caused by consecutive dissection of the ligaments from anterior to posterior: dissection of the bifurcate ligament leads to a significant increase of plantarflexion and dorsiflexion (*P* = .028). Dissection of the IER resulted in a significant increase of eversion and inversion (*P* = .046). Additional dissection of the LTCL was followed by a significant increase of internal and external rotation (*P* = .028). (*C*) Increasing subtalar instability caused by consecutive dissection of the ligament from posterior to anterior: dissection of the CFL leads to a significant change of overall joint kinematics; it alters all motion directions in the subtalar joint. Thus, it develops a relevant subtalar instability (*P* = .028). BL, bifurcate ligament; NA, native condition. (*From* Weindel S, Schmidt R, Rammelt S, et al. Subtalar instability: a biomechanical cadaver study. Arch Orthop Trauma Surg 2010;130:313–9, with permission.)

and sensory neuropathies may predispose to STI. Bonnel and colleagues[24] pointed to the role of hindfoot deformity as a trigger for CAI and STI.

Deltoid and spring ligament insufficiency has been categorized by Hintermann and colleagues[20,34] into 3 types, with type 1 lesions occurring proximally at the anterior colliculus of the medial malleolus, type 2 lesions corresponding with intermediate deltoid lesions, and type 3 lesions corresponding with an involvement of the distal deltoid and the spring ligament. The more universal classification of peritalar instability comprises the 2 main deformity types of valgus and varus deformity, with each group including subgroups resulting in a total of 9 valgus and varus deformity subtypes.[10]

CLINICAL PRESENTATION AND ASSESSMENT
History and Clinical Examination

The difficulty in differentiating acute ankle instability and STI has been stated by several investigators.[3–5,7] Lateral swelling, ecchymosis, and tenderness may be present during palpation at the acute stage but are unspecific. The value of any clinical stress test after acute trauma is limited by the patient's pain and muscular counteraction. In general, patients with STI do not present to the clinician after a single traumatic event.[7] Frequently, those patients have similar complaints as in CAI. Some report an inversion injury, which is common for both ankle and subtalar joint sprains and does not allow any discrimination between these entities.[12] Many patients report a feeling of giving way or rolling over, in particular on uneven ground, which becomes pronounced with increased physical activity.[4] Some individuals project their pain to the sinus tarsi and the lateral hindfoot.[7,12] Patients with STI prefer to wear high-top shoes or stabilizing orthotics,[11,35] in contrast with patients with CAI, who prefer flat-top shoes.[4]

A specific test for chronic STI is the anterolateral drawer test, in which a combined inversion, internal rotation, and adduction stress is applied to the forefoot while the hindfoot is held by the examiner in maximum extension (dorsiflexion) in order to block the inadvertent motion at the ankle level[3–5,36] (**Fig. 3**). A positive test reveals an increased anterior and medial shift as well as a varus tilt of the calcaneus beneath the talus. The relevance and validity of this test have been validated in a cadaver model using selective ligament transection and direct measurement of increased instability diagnostic in which a 4-mm threshold provided 100% sensitivity and 67% specificity with excellent intraobserver reproducibility.[37] To detect any static deformity at the hindfoot or lower leg (eg, a cavovarus deformity), the patient should routinely be examined while standing, which has particularly been recommended for examination of chronic medial instability at the ankle and subtalar joint.[20,21] Furthermore, the Coleman block test should be performed to reveal any forefoot-driven hindfoot deformity. The variable symptoms of sinus tarsi syndrome, which represent a conglomerate of heterogeneous clinical entities more than a diagnosis, are observed in some patients with chronic STI.[26,38,39] Sinus tarsi syndrome has been linked to scarring of the ITCL in arthroscopic studies.[4,40,41] An injection test into the sinus tarsi with local anesthetics can be helpful to further localize the source of pain, especially when the pain cannot be attributed to any anatomic structure.[26]

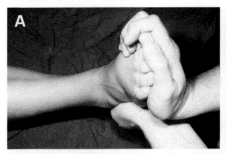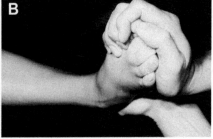

Fig. 3. (*A*) Clinical testing of anterolateral rotational instability. The ankle joint is blocked in extension with the right hand of the examiner (*B*) while the left hand induces a varus tilt of the hindfoot. (*From* Zwipp H, Rammelt S. Ligamente: Rupturen und Luxationen. In: Zwipp H, Rammelt S, editors. Tscherne Unfallchirurgie. Heidelberg (Germany): Springer; 2014. p. 215–70; with permission.)

Radiographic Examination

Plain anteroposterior and lateral radiographs of the ankle and hindfoot may show bony avulsions at the subtalar joint from acute or chronic ligamentous injuries. Frequently, avulsions or rounded ossicles are found along Hellpap's[41] fracture line of supination, ranging from the ankle across the subtalar and calcaneocuboid joint down to the tuberosity of the fifth metatarsal.[4,41]

There has been a long-standing and controversial discussion about the value of stress radiography to detect and quantify STI.[3–5,7,33,39,42,43] There is no doubt that the 3D motion that occurs during subtalar joint motion is difficult to see in two-dimensional radiographs. Some of the recommended techniques might at least be beneficial to support the clinical impression of STI. The techniques described by Zwipp and Krettek,[44] and later by Ishii and colleagues,[42] resemble the anterolateral drawer test recommended for clinical evaluation[3,4,36] with the ankle held in dorsiflexion and forefoot supinated. The shift of the lateral talar process in relation to the subtalar joint facet yields a relative measure that has been tested in cadavers with sequential sectioning of the CFL and ITCL, healthy probands, and patients with STI.[42] Although hand-held stress testing is impaired by the variability of stress exerted by individual examiners, the application of a device with defined force allows for better standardized testing conditions (**Fig. 4**). The Telos device (METAX Inc, Hungen-Obbornhofen, Germany), which was originally developed for assessment of ligamentous ankle instability, can be applied for subtalar stress testing.[3,4,44]

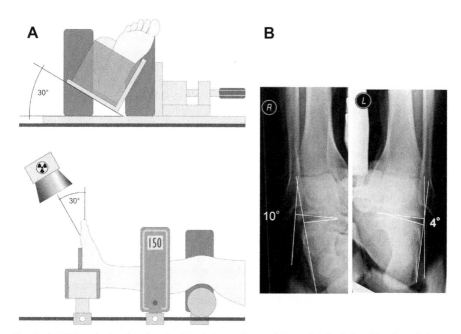

Fig. 4. (A) Telos device for standardized stress views of the subtalar joint. The foot is internally rotated for 30°, the x-ray beam is tilted plantarward 30°. The applied force is limited to 150 N. (B) Clinical example of a patient with chronic subtalar joint instability of the right side, in which a talocalcaneal tilt of 10°, a talocalcaneal angle of 15°, and a medial shift of the talus of 6 mm can be measured. The left subtalar joint is intact. (*From* Mittlmeier T, Wichelhaus A. Subtalar joint instability. Eur J Trauma Emerg Surg 2015;41:624; with permission.)

The radiographs resemble the Brodén views of the subtalar joint. With a varus force of 150 N applied to the hindfoot, a talocalcaneal angle of less than 10°, a talocalcaneal tilt of less than 5°, and a medial offset of the talus of less than 5° are considered normal[3,4] (see **Fig. 4**). In unilateral instability, comparison with the contralateral intact side allows for the exclusion of ligamentous laxity and thus false-positive test results.[32,45] A difference in talocalcaneal tilt of greater than 5° speaks in favor of STI.[44,45] Radiographic modifications such as digital tomosynthesis can help to improve the image quality and to better read out the quantitative values of instability,[46,47] but they still lack a 3D view of the subtalar joint. Therefore, Lee and colleagues[39] recently compared 3 variants of manual stress testing for STI in which the test, which imitated the clinical anterolateral stress test, was shown to have the highest degree of intrarater and interrater reproducibility. In addition, a significantly increased talar rotation compared with the uninjured side was observed in 66 patients with injuries to the AFTL and CFL. With additional injury to the cervical ligament (OTCL), a significantly higher increment of talar rotation was seen in 19 patients detected via MRI and surgical exploration.[39]

Three-Dimensional Imaging

Kinematic ankle CT scanning with interactive reconstruction during dynamic exposures in a full pronation and supination cycle allows for a spatial and functional analysis of subtalar joint motion.[30] However, the value of CT imaging has been questioned because the ligaments cannot be visualized directly, and stress MRI has been reported to better reflect the 3D motion at the subtalar joint, as shown in cadaver specimens more than 12 years ago.[44] In a more recent clinical study in 72 clinically stable ankle joints and 28 ankles with CAI, the use of an MRI-compatible stress device in 1-T open MRI was helpful to visualize directly both the ligaments and the 3D motion, including that of the subtalar joint.[31] The investigators further performed a correlation analysis with clinical scores and emphasized the clear-cut discrimination between the stable and unstable ankle/subtalar joints, including subjects with functional and mechanical instability.[31] With the use of 3D isotropic high-resolution MRI with a dedicated coil for the ankle joint, the dimensions of the subtalar ligament components (ATCL, OTCL, ITCL, CFL, AFTL) can be measured directly.[32] The investigators found significantly smaller dimensions of the ATCL in 23 patients with chronic subtalar instability compared with normals matched for sex, age, body weight, and height but did not see any differences in the geometry of the ITCL, CFL, or ATFL between patients and controls. Based on a receiver operator characteristic analysis of the ATCL dimensions, a cutoff of 2.1 mm for ATCL thickness had a sensitivity of 66.7% and a specificity of 66.7% (area under the curve [AUC] = 0.765; $P = .007$) for the diagnosis of STI, whereas a cutoff of 7.9 mm for ATCL width had a sensitivity of 80.0% and a specificity of 76.2% (AUC = 0.778; $P = .005$) to distinguish patients with STI from controls.[32]

An alternative to radiographic techniques might be stress ultrasonography examination, which is limited in its validity by the dependence on the experience of the individual examiner.[11]

Subtalar Arthroscopy

Apart from all these noninvasive test approaches, subtalar joint arthroscopy has been advocated as valuable diagnostic tool, in particular in cases in which the working diagnosis of a sinus tarsi syndrome was inconclusive for a further differentiation and assignment to a distinct diagnosis.[39,40,43] Subtalar joint arthroscopy is rarely indicated as a stand-alone procedure[43,48,49] but can be embedded into the diagnostic algorithm as an intraoperative decision-making step before ligamentous reconstruction.[32,39,43,50]

In summary, STI can be diagnosed clinically when 4 of the 5 following criteria are fulfilled[32,50]:

1. Recurrent ankle/hindfoot sprains
2. Sinus tarsi syndrome and tenderness
3. Hindfoot laxity or giving way
4. Hindfoot instability during clinical examination
5. Hindfoot instability in stress radiographs

High-resolution MRI of the ankle and subtalar joints can then represent a further logical step for identifying and differentiating the amount of ligamentous injury before a decision is made for surgical reconstruction. Intraoperatively, dynamic fluoroscopy and subtalar joint arthroscopy can then be conducted to visualize subtalar joint laxity and synovitis, and to diagnose associated ligamentous injuries.[32,50,51]

Patients with chronic ligamentous lesions at the medial ankle and the subtalar joint may present with flatfoot, pronounced valgus, and pronation of the affected foot.[20] In contrast with patients with a posterior tibial tendon dysfunction, those patients with STI are able to actively correct hindfoot deformity and perform a single heel rise. With associated hindfoot and midfoot deformities, weight-bearing radiographs are preferred to stress radiographs. An additional MRI scan might help to identify a ligamentous lesion at the medial malleolus, osteochondral lesions, or a disorder of the spring ligament and the tibialis posterior tendon.[20,52] The value of intraoperative stress fluoroscopy and arthroscopy has been emphasized in relation to the recommendations given for lateral ankle instability.[20]

TREATMENT OF SUBTALAR JOINT INSTABILITY
Acute Injury

The recommended treatment of acute combined ligamentous lesions of the ankle and subtalar joint becoming manifest as anterolateral rotational instability is equivalent to that of injuries that are limited to the lateral collateral ankle ligaments.[3,4,36] Depending on the initial amount of edema and swelling a non–weight-bearing split lower leg cast is applied until swelling subsides. The treatment of choice is functional with application of an ankle-foot-orthosis, which limits supination and can be worn within the patient's own shoe with pain-adapted full weight bearing.[3,4] The positive effect of a semirigid ankle brace on both the ankle and the subtalar joint regarding the limitation of inversion has been proved in biomechanical trials.[35,53] The orthosis is worn for 6 weeks, followed by a course of proprioceptive training and strengthening of the peroneal muscles in order to avoid recurrent sprains and functional instability.[4]

Chronic Subtalar Joint Instability

Patients with chronic STI are examined for proprioceptive deficits. Typically, a chronic functional instability warrants a defined period of proprioceptive training, including sensomotoric taping, stretching of the triceps surae, and prescription of insoles or wedging of the lateral shoe.[3,4,53] In case of failure after a period of continuous exercises of 12 to 16 weeks' duration, surgical treatment should be considered depending on the clinical symptoms and the frequency of ankle and/or subtalar sprains.[3,4] Any kind of hindfoot malalignment should be traded off against the concomitant role of ligamentous components of instability.[8] Even simultaneous correction of osseous and ligamentous components of instability represents a viable option to avoid a failure or recurrence of instability.

In general, anatomic repair should be given the preference rather than nonanatomic reconstruction.[3,4,11,54,55] If CAI and STI coexist, the reconstruction of the CFL seems to be of paramount importance for restoration of stability.[3,4,55] In case of dystopic malunion and elongation of the CFL, an adequate shortening and transosseous refixation of the CFL, optionally with the inclusion of a bone block from the distal insertional area, can be performed[3,4,54,55] (**Fig. 5**). In case of poor consistency of the remnants of the CFL, a doubled and distally pedicled periosteal flap can be used to augment the reconstructed CFL (**Fig. 6**). Another augmentation option could be performed with the help of the distal extensor retinaculum.[56] A modification of the Broström-Gould technique using a tenodesis with allograft significantly decreased subtalar and ankle inversion and subtalar internal rotation compared with the unstable condition in chronic STI, but the tenodesis was unable to restore subtalar and ankle inversion compared with the intact state.[57] Saragaglia and colleagues[58] introduced a modification of the Broström-Gould technique that particularly reinforces the OTCL by mobilization of a rectangular flap of the superior section of the IER of 1 cm by 3 to 4 cm width, which remains pedicled at the calcaneal side near the entrance to the sinus tarsi. Thereafter, an L-shaped capsulotomy and inspection of the subtalar and lateral ankle joint is performed for visualizing any additional cartilaginous lesions and identification of the remnants of the ATFL, CFL, and the sinus tarsi.[59] In addition, a periosteal flap pedicled at the distal fibula can be used to reinforce the anterior capsular reinsertion before closure. The residual capsule-ligament complex and its extensor retinaculum reinforcement are reinserted onto the anterior part and tip of the lateral malleolus with 1 anchor holding the capsule, another anchor holding the anterior tibiofibular and CFLs, and the extensor

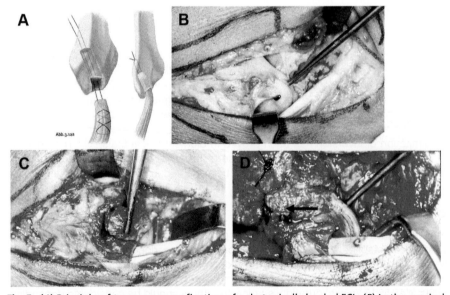

Fig. 5. (*A*) Principle of transosseous refixation of a dystopically healed FCL. (*B*) In the surgical field a dystopically healed and elongated FCL (*C*) is elevated with a small bone chip. The bone chip is advanced proximally (*arrow*) within a trough made in the distal fibula (*D*), which tensions the elongated ligament.

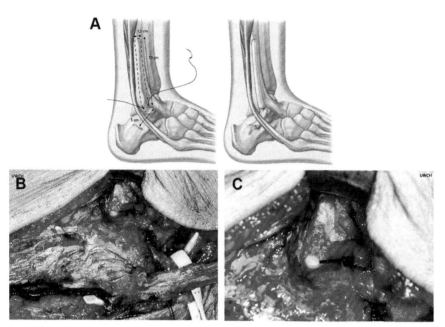

Fig. 6. (*A*) Principle of FCL augmentation via an autologous periosteal flap that is mobilized over a length of 10 cm and a width of 1.5 cm and pedicled at the distal fibula (*B*) where it crosses under the peroneal tendons to reinforce the chronically weakened FCL. (*C*) The periosteal flap is doubled over the FCL and sutured in itself. (*From* Zwipp H, Rammelt S. Ligamente: Rupturen und Luxationen. In: Zwipp H, Rammelt S, editors. Tscherne Unfallchirurgie. Heidelberg (Germany): Springer; 2014. p. 215–70; with permission.)

retinaculum flap being fixed with an interference screw between the two. The sutures are tied with the foot in a neutral, slightly everted position. The periosteal flap is sutured onto the lateral aspect of the fibular malleolus, reinforcing the reconstruction. Further sutures, holding the extensor digitorum brevis muscle, completely close the sinus tarsi entry (**Fig. 7**).

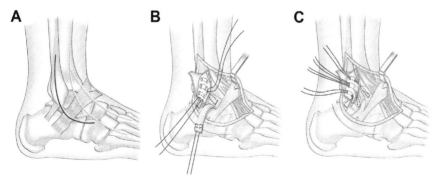

Fig. 7. Anatomic repair including IER reinforcement. (*A*) Approach. (*B*) IER harvesting. (*C*) Reinsertion of genuine ligament bundles and reinforcement. (*Reproduced from* Tourné Y, Mabit C. Lateral ligament reconstruction procedures of the ankle. Orthop Traumatol Surg Res 2017;103:S171–81; Elsevier Masson SAS. All rights reserved.)

Apart from these widespread techniques primarily developed for CAI, information about the replacement or augmentation of any ligamentous components of the sinus tarsi are scarce. Historically, the first attempts for treatment of STI were tenodesis techniques representing modifications of the Elmslie procedure using one-half of the distally pedicled peroneus brevis tendon, which in turn sacrifices an essential active evertor of the foot.[5,7] The Chrisman-Snook tenodesis has gained wider acceptance and has been further modified[60] (**Fig. 8**A). All nonanatomic reconstruction techniques have a substantial inherent risk of subtalar stiffness and a consecutive long-term risk of developing secondary osteoarthritis.[4,5,7]

Anatomic reconstruction techniques of the ITCL were recommended early[25,26,33] using a strip of the Achilles tendon or the anterior half of the peroneus brevis tendon (**Fig. 8**B). These investigators pointed out that the identification of the correct insertion points and the positioning of the graft may be difficult in an open technique. Therefore, proposals for an arthroscopically guided technique have been made with suture anchors, staples, or endobuttons being used for graft fixation (**Fig. 8**C). From the present perspective, most of those techniques addressed the replacement of the ATCL, neglecting most other ligamentous stabilizers of the subtalar joint. Recently, a technique has been published that incorporates the simultaneous reconstruction of the ITCL, the OTCL, and the CFL[45,50] (**Fig. 8**D). The authors' preferred treatment of STI consists of repair of the interosseous and cervical ligaments with one-half of the

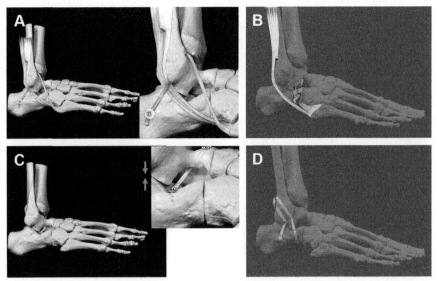

Fig. 8. (*A*) Principle of extra-anatomic reconstruction of chronic subtalar joint instability using a pedicled tendon autograft from the peroneus brevis tendon in a modified Elmslie ligamentoplasty. (*B*) Principle of reconstruction of chronic subtalar joint instability via a pedicled peroneus brevis tendon autograft to replace the ITCL. (*C*) Principle of reconstruction of chronic subtalar joint instability with a free hamstrings tendon autograft in a purely arthroscopically guided technique to replace the ITCL using an endobutton and suture anchor system or staples to fix the graft. (*D*) Principle of reconstruction of chronic subtalar joint instability with a semitendinosus tendon allograft to address the OTCL, ITCL, and the CFL in an arthroscopically guided technique with triple interference screw fixation. (*Data from* Refs.[25,26,45,59]; *From* Mittlmeier T, Wichelhaus A. Subtalar joint instability. Eur J Trauma Emerg Surg 2015;41:627; with permission.)

peroneus longus tendon in order to avoid relevant donor morbidity (ie, weakened eversion) and achieve a near-anatomic reconstruction (**Fig. 9**).

OUTCOME

In contrast with the postulated frequency of STI, the number of reports about surgical reconstruction in STI is limited.[1,2,9,25,26,33,36,60–63] The main results are summarized in **Table 1**. Most studies are retrospective cumulative case series with limited numbers of patients included and variable follow-up periods. Consequently, the evidence level of all those reports is low (exclusively level IV and V). Despite general recommendations for anatomic reconstruction, the results of both nonanatomic and anatomic techniques seem to be similar. The risk portfolio comprises intraoperative lesions of cutaneous nerves as the intermediate branch of the superficial peroneal nerve or the terminal branch of the sural nerve, postoperative subtalar joint stiffness, recurrent instability, or secondary osteoarthritis. Isolated subtalar arthrodesis has been proposed as a preferable treatment option in case of persistent STI and subtalar osteoarthritis.[64]

The evidence for medial STI is even more sparse. Medial STI can rarely be addressed by isolated ligamentous reconstruction to achieve long-term peritalar stability without, in particular, the progressive development of osteoarthritis.[10] Osseous balancing by realignment procedures has been recommended, which comprise supramalleolar and inframalleolar osteotomies.[10,21] For dynamic

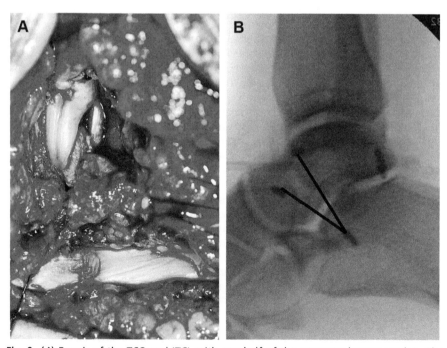

Fig. 9. (A) Repair of the TCO and ITCL with one-half of the peroneus longus tendon. The bone tunnels are drilled in a V shape through the talar neck in order to obtain a near-anatomic reconstruction. The free tendon graft is fixed with suture anchors. The CFL is re-attached to the tip of the fibula with another suture anchor. (B) The V-shaped course of the tendon graft.

Table 1
Outcome following surgical treatment of subtalar joint instability

Author and Year	Technique	Number of Patients (n)	Excellent or Good Results (%)
Larsen,[9] 1988	PB	25	93
Chrisman & Snook,[60] 1969	PB	3	100
Schon et al,[62] 1991	Modified Elmslie	NS	NS
Pisani,[25] 1996; Pisani et al,[26] 2005	ITCL anatomic	47	91
Karlsson et al,[2] 1998	Anatomic + IER reinforcement	22	82
Kato,[33] 1995	ITCL or triligamentous	14 (2*/12#)	>90
Thermann et al,[36] 1997	Chrisman-Snook	34	91
Liu et al,[48] 2011	Hamstrings autograft	1	(100)
Jung et al,[50] 2015	Anatomic ITCL, OTCL, and FCL	20	100

Abbreviations: NS, not stated; PB, pedicled peroneus brevis graft.

planovalgus deformity resulting from ruptures of the spring ligament, a combination of osseous and ligamentous procedures are recommended.[52]

SUMMARY

The complex anatomy of the subtalar joint continues to be a source of misunderstanding. The debate about STI should not be limited to the ligamentous components, which contribute to lateral stability, because the ITCL, parts of the deltoid ligament, and the ligaments of the TCN joint essentially account for medial subtalar joint stability. The function of the subtalar joint is intrinsically linked to the function of the ankle joint, with mutual compensation mechanisms that are still not well understood. Despite its presumably high prevalence after inversion injuries, STI seems to be a diagnosis that is often missed initially and mostly becomes apparent clinically at a later stage of chronic STI. The diagnosis should be based on an algorithm that includes clinical, functional, and imaging parameters to create a sound basis for decision making and selection of the proper treatment. Surgical reconstruction techniques addressing ankle or combined ankle/subtalar instability, including a repair of the CFL with reinforcement via a periosteal flap or an advancement of parts of the IER, seem to be effective to restore both ankle and subtalar joint stability. It is still a matter of discussion when and how isolated or combined ligamentous and osseous procedures to supply subtalar stability should be performed. Most of these procedures address the reconstruction of isolated ligamentous components of the sinus and canalis tarsi and nonanatomic procedures are still advocated. Future research should focus on the analysis of 3D motion at the ankle and subtalar joint under physiologic and pathologic conditions, the corresponding interplay, and the spatial effects of any reconstruction mode.

REFERENCES

1. Karlsson J, Eriksson BI, Renström PA. Subtalar ankle instability. A review. Sports Med 1997;24:337–46.
2. Karlsson J, Eriksson BI, Renström P. Subtalar instability of the foot. A review and results after surgical treatment. Scand J Med Sci Sports 1998;8:191–7.
3. Zwipp H. Chirurgie des Fußes. Wien (Austria): Springer; 1994.

4. Zwipp H, Rammelt S. Ligamente: Rupturen und Luxationen. In: Zwipp H, Rammelt S, editors. Tscherne Unfallchirurgie. Fuß. Heidelberg (Germany): Springer; 2014. p. 215–70.

5. Aynardi S, Pedowitz DI, Raikin SM. Subtalar instability. Foot Ankle Clin 2015;20: 243–52.

6. Weindel S, Schmidt R, Rammelt S, et al. Subtalar instability: a biomechanical cadaver study. Arch Orthop Trauma Surg 2010;130:313–9.

7. Keefe DT, Haddad SL. Subtalar instability. Etiology, diagnosis, and management. Foot Ankle Clin 2002;7:577–609.

8. Usuelli FG, Mason L, Grassi M, et al. Lateral and hindfoot instability: a new clinical based classification. Foot Ankle Surg 2014;20:231–6.

9. Larsen E. Tendon transfer for lateral ankle and subtalar joint instability. Acta Orthop Scand 1988;59:168–72.

10. Hintermann B, Knupp M, Barg A. Peritalar instability. Foot Ankle Int 2012;33: 450–4.

11. Barg A, Tochigi Y, Amendola A, et al. Subtalar instability: diagnosis and treatment. Foot Ankle Int 2012;33:151–60.

12. Mittlmeier T, Wichelhaus A. Subtalar joint instability. Eur J Trauma Emerg Surg 2015;41:623–9.

13. Michels F, Perreira H, Calder J, et al. Searching for consensus in the approach to patients with chronic lateral ankle instability: ask the expert. Knee Surg Sports Traumatol Arthrosc 2017. https://doi.org/10.1007/s00167-017-4556-0.

14. Bartoníček J, Rammelt S, Naňka O. Anatomy of the subtalar joint. Foot Ankle Clin, in press.

15. Inman VT. The joints of the ankle. Baltimore (MD): Williams & Wilkins; 1976.

16. Sarrafian SK. Biomechanics of the subtalar joint complex. Clin Orthop Relat Res 1993;290:17–26.

17. Wood-Jones F. The talocalcaneal articulation. Lancet 1944;24:241–2.

18. Choisne J, Ringleb S, Samaan MA, et al. Influence of kinematic analysis methods on detecting ankle and subtalar joint instability. J Biomech 2012;45:46–52.

19. Poonja AJ, Hirano M, Khakimov D, et al. Anatomical study of the cervical and interosseous talocalcaneal ligaments of the foot with surgical relevance. Cureus 2017;9:e1382.

20. Lötscher P, Lang TH, Zwicky L, et al. Osteoligamentous injuries of the medial ankle joint. Eur J Trauma Emerg Surg 2015;41:615–21.

21. Krähenbühl N, Horn-Lang T, Hintermann B, et al. The subtalar joint: a complex mechanism. EFORT Open Rev 2017;2:309–16.

22. Pellegrini MJ, Glisson RR, Wurm M, et al. Systematic quantification of stabilizing effects of subtalar joint soft-tissue constraints in a novel cadaveric model. J Bone Joint Surg Am 2016;98:842–8.

23. Tochigi Y, Amendola A, Rudert M, et al. The role of the interosseous talocalcaneal ligament in subtalar joint instability. Foot Ankle Int 2004;25:588–96.

24. Bonnel F, Toullec E, Mabit C, et al. Chronic ankle instability: biomechanics and pathomechanics of ligaments injury and associated lesions. Orthop Traumatol Surg Res 2010;96:424–32.

25. Pisani G. Chronic laxity of the subtalar joint. Orthopedics 1996;19:431–7.

26. Pisani G, Pisani PC, Parino E. Sinus tarsi syndrome and subtalar joint instability. Clin Podiatr Med Surg 2005;22:63–77.

27. Beimers L, Juijthof GJM, Blankevoort L, et al. In-vivo range of motion of the subtalar joint using computed tomography. J Biomech 2008;41:1390–7.

28. Pearce TJ, Buckley RE. Subtalar joint movement: clinical and computed tomography scan correlation. Foot Ankle Int 1999;20:428–32.

29. Roach KE, Foreman KB, Barg A, et al. Application of high-speed dual fluoroscopy to study in vivo tibiotalar and subtalar kinematics in patients with chronic ankle instability and asymptomatic control subjects during dynamic activities. Foot Ankle Int 2017;38:1–13.

30. Teixeira PAG, Formery A-S, Jacquot A, et al. Quantitative analysis of subtalar joint motion with 4D CT: proof of concept with cadaveric and healthy subject evaluation. AJR Am J Roentgenol 2016;208:150–8.

31. Seebauer CJ, Bail HJ, Rump JC, et al. Ankle laxity: stress investigation under MRI control. AJR Am J Roentgenol 2013;201:496–504.

32. Kim TH, Moon SG, Jung H-G, et al. Subtalar instability: imaging features of subtalar ligaments on 3D isotropic ankle MRI. BMC Musculoskelet Disord 2017; 18:475.

33. Kato T. The diagnosis and treatment of instability of the subtalar joint. J Bone Joint Surg Br 1995;77:400–6.

34. Hintermann B, Valderrabano V, Boss A, et al. Medial ankle instability: an exploratory, prospective study of fifty-two cases. Am J Sports Med 2004;32:183–90.

35. Choisne J, Hoch MC, Bawab S, et al. The effects of a semi-rigid ankle brace on a simulated isolated subtalar joint instability. J Orthop Res 2013;31:1869–75.

36. Thermann H, Zwipp H, Tscherne H. Treatment algorithm of chronic ankle and subtalar instability. Foot Ankle Int 1997;18:163–9.

37. Vaseenon T, Gao Y, Phisitkul P. Comparison of two manual tests for ankle laxity due to rupture of the lateral ankle ligaments. Iowa Orthop J 2012;32:9–16.

38. Helgeson K. Examination and intervention for sinus tarsi syndrome. North Am J Sports Phys Ther 2009;4:29–37.

39. Lee BH, Choi K-H, Seo DY. Diagnostic validity of alternative manual stress radiographic technique detecting subtalar instability with concomitant ankle instability. Knee Surg Sports Traumatol Arthrosc 2016;24:1029–39.

40. Frey C, Feder KS, DiGiovanni C. Arthroscopic evaluation of the subtalar joint: does sinus tarsi syndrome exist? Foot Ankle Int 1999;20:185–91.

41. Hellpap W. Das vernachlässigte untere Sprunggelenk. Die "Frakturlinie der Supination". Arch Orthop Unfallchir 1963;55:289–300.

42. Ishii T, Miyagawa S, Fukubayashi T, et al. Subtalar stress radiography under forced dorsiflexion and supination. J Bone Joint Surg Br 1996;78:56–60.

43. Lee KB, Bai LB, Song EK, et al. Subtalar arthroscopy for sinus tarsi syndrome: arthroscopic findings and clinical outcome of 33 consecutive cases. Arthroscopy 2008;24:1130–4.

44. Zwipp H, Krettek C. Diagnostik und Therapie der akuten und chronischen Bandinstabilität des unteren Sprunggelenkes. Orthopade 1986;15:472–8 [in German].

45. Jung HG, Kim TH. Subtalar instability reconstruction with an allograft: technical note. Foot Ankle Int 2012;33:682–5.

46. Teramoto A, Watanabe K, Takashima H, et al. Subtalar joint stress imaging with tomosynthesis. Foot Ankle Spec 2014;7:182–4.

47. Ringleb SI, Udupa JK, Siegler S, et al. The effect of ankle ligament damage and surgical reconstruction on the mechanics of the ankle and subtalar joints revealed by three-dimensional stress MRI. J Orthop Res 2005;23:743–9.

48. Liu C, Jiao C, Hu Y. Interosseous talocalcaneal ligament reconstruction with hamstrings autograft under subtalar arthroscopy: case report. Foot Ankle Int 2011;32: 1089–94.

49. Oloff LM, Schulhoger SD, Bocko AP. Subtalar joint arthroscopy for sinus tarsi syndrome: a review of 20 cases. J Foot Ankle Surg 2001;40:152–7.
50. Jung HG, Park JT, Shin MH, et al. Outcome of subtalar instability reconstruction using the semitendinosus allograft tendon and biotenodesis screws. Knee Surg Sports Traumatol Arthrosc 2015;23:2376–83.
51. Sugimoto K, Isomoto S, Samoto N, et al. Recent developments in the treatment of ankle and subtalar instability. Open Orthop J 2017;11(Suppl 4):687–96.
52. Steginsky B, Vora A. What to do with the spring ligament. Foot Ankle Clin 2017;22: 515–27.
53. Kobayashi T, Saka M, Suzuki E, et al. The effects of a semi-rigid brace or taping on talocrural and subtalar kinematics in chronic ankle instability. Foot Ankle Spec 2014;7:471–7.
54. Tourné Y, Mabit C, Moroney PJ, et al. Long-term follow-up of lateral reconstruction with extensor retinaculum flap for chronic ankle instability. Foot Ankle Int 2012;33: 1079–86.
55. Tourné Y, Mabit C. Lateral ligament reconstruction procedures of the ankle. Orthop Traumatol Surg Res 2017;103:S171–81.
56. Gould N, Seligson D, Gassman J. Early and late repair of lateral ligament of the ankle. Foot Ankle 1980;1:84–9.
57. Choisne J, Hoch MC, Alexander I, et al. Effect of direct ligament repair and tenodesis reconstruction on simulated subtalar joint instability. Foot Ankle Int 2017;38: 324–30.
58. Saragaglia D, Fontanel F, Montbarbon E, et al. Reconstruction for the lateral ankle ligaments using an inferior extensor retinaculum flap. Foot Ankle Int 1997;18: 723–5.
59. Trichine F, Friha T, Boukabou A, et al. Surgical treatment of lateral ankle instability using an inferior extensor retinaculum flap: a retrospective study. J Foot Ankle Surg 2018;57(2):226–31.
60. Chrisman OD, Snook GA. Reconstruction of lateral ligament tears of the ankle. An experimental study and clinical evaluation of seven patients treated with a new modification of the Elmslie procedure. J Bone Joint Surg Am 1969;51:904–12.
61. Castaing J, Falaise B, Burdin P. Ligamentoplasty using the peroneus brevis in the treatment of chronic instabilities of the ankle. Long-term review. Orthop Traumatol Surg Res 2014;100:33–5.
62. Schon LC, Clanton TO, Baxter DE. Reconstruction for subtalar instability: a review. Foot Ankle 1991;11:319–25.
63. Acevedo JI, Myerson MS. Modification of the Chrisman-Snook technique. Foot Ankle Int 2000;21:154–5.
64. Mann RA, Beaman DN, Horton GA. Isolated subtalar arthrodesis. Foot Ankle Int 1998;19:511–9.

Arthroereisis
What Have We Learned?

Cristian A. Ortiz, MD[a],*, Emilio Wagner, MD[b], Pablo Wagner, MD[b]

KEYWORDS

- Flatfoot • Treatment • Surgery • Arthroereisis • Pedriatrics • Adults

KEY POINTS

- The techniques used to correct flatfoot deformity can be grouped into 3 categories: soft tissue, bone (osteotomies and arthrodesis), and arthroereisis.
- Arthroereisis procedures were originally designed for pediatric treatment and generally involve joint-sparing techniques that correct the flatfoot deformity while preserving foot function.
- Different kinds of arthroereisis procedures are described, including sinus tarsi implants, tarsi canal implants, and calcaneo stop.
- Arthroereisis is a minimally invasive procedure performed near the apex of flatfeet deformity in a constrained structure.
- Arthroereisis can be performed alone or as a complementary procedure to correct flatfoot.

 Video content accompanies this article at http://www.foot.theclinics.com.

INTRODUCTION

Flatfoot is a common deformity in adult and pediatric populations, with a 5% incidence. The deformity is characterized by a reduction or absence of the medial arch, medial protrusion of the talar head, and valgus hindfoot under weight-bearing conditions.[1,2] The deformity can be symptomatic or asymptomatic, flexible or rigid.[3] Clinical evaluation must include an assessment for the presence of subtalar or midtarsal synostosis, ligamentous laxity, stiffness, concomitant deformities, Achilles tendon shortening, and so forth. Patients should be examined completely including a proper gait analysis. Patients who are not able to compensate for the deformity during walking and who keep their feet in permanent pronation usually are symptomatic earlier.

Imaging should begin with full weight-bearing radiographs.[4,5] Special attention should be pointed to ask patients not to correct the deformity when the radiographs

Disclosure Statement: The authors have nothing to disclose.
[a] Foot and Ankle Department, Clinica Universidad de los Andes, Universidad del, Santiago, Chile; [b] Foot and Ankle Department, Clinica Alemana, Universidad del Desarrollo, Avenida la Plaza 2501, Santiago 7620001, Chile
* Corresponding author. Colina del Sur 9779, Vitacura 5951, Santiago RM 7600976, Chile.
E-mail address: caortizm@gmail.com

Foot Ankle Clin N Am 23 (2018) 415–434
https://doi.org/10.1016/j.fcl.2018.04.010
1083-7515/18/© 2018 Elsevier Inc. All rights reserved.

are taken, because the authors have observed confusing conclusions when patients with flexible deformities unintentionally start to correct the flatfoot deformity as they do at rest at the end of the day.

Most symptomatic patients get significant relief when using inserts (off the shelf or custom made).[6]

When conservative treatment does not allow patients to come back to normal life, including daily day activities, moderate physical exercise, basic shoe wear, and so forth, surgical treatment should be considered.[7]

Although indications and surgical treatment are still under debate, different treatment options have been recommended for flatfoot deformity, including soft tissue procedures, osteotomies, arthrodesis, and recently arthroereisis (**Box 1**). The last option has become more popular due to the high success rates reported in Europe, South America, and Asia. It was initially described for children, but increasing indications are expanding even in adults. This has led clinicians to put more attention to indications, technique, rehabilitation, and potential complications.[8,9]

RATIONALE FOR ARTHROEREISIS

Arthroereisis procedures were originally designed for the treatment of pediatric deformities and generally involved joint-sparing techniques, that is, correction of the flatfoot while preserving foot function.[10] Regardless of the implant design or material, the rationale for this procedure is that placing a calcaneal motion locking device into the sinus tarsi or tarsal canal restores and maintains the physiologic alignment between the talus and calcaneus during bone remodeling while correcting the deformity before it turns into a rigid one. Apparently, these locking devices do not negatively affect the biomechanics of the subtalar joint or alter the normal closed kinetic chain mechanics while limiting excessive hindfoot pronation.[11]

Historically, arthroereisis was first described by Grice in 1952[12] for correction of paralytic flatfeet in children without affecting foot growth. Several complications were observed, such as loss of correction or overcorrection. Haraldsson[13] and Lelievere[14] first described the possibility of blocking the sinus tarsi, restricting subtalar motion but avoiding fusions. Lelievre introduced the term, *lateral arthroereisis*, for a temporary staple across the subtalar joint. Batchelor modified the technique with the introduction of a fibular peg blindly inserted through the sinus tarsi. A high nonunion rate, however, was observed.[15]

Box 1
Surgical options for flatfoot deformity

Soft tissue procedures
  Achilles tendon lengthening
  Kidner procedure
  Spring ligament repair

Osteotomies
  Medializing calcaneal osteotomy
  Lateral column lengthening (Evans)
  Z osteotomy

Artrodesis
  Triple arthrodesis
  Double arthrodesis (subtalar and talonavicular)

Arthroereisis

Subotnick[16] first described a sinus tarsi implant consisting of a block of silicone elastomer. But Viladot[7] was first to describe a true sinus tarsi implant. In Viladot's study, a success rate of 99% in 234 patients was shown using a cup-shaped silicone implant.[7]

In 1995 Alvarez[17] published on the calcaneo-stop technique, limiting motion in the subtalar joint through a screw inserted into the calcaneus using the sinus tarsi as the entry point. The same principle was used but with a screw placed in the talus to block the subtalar joint. Good results were shown in 475 cases with long follow-up, up to 112 months.

Even after implant removal, correction remains maintained over time.[18]

TYPES OF ARTHROEREISIS

Since its first description by Grice, various types of arthroereisis have been developed and used. Some of them have stood the test of time; others have been abandoned. Vogler[19] classified implant for the subtalar joint into 3 types (**Table 1**).

Although there are no studies comparing the different types of arthroereisis implants, the authors have observed some important facts that may aid in the decision-making process. In the authors' experience, a higher extrusion rate of the classis sinus tarsi implants compared with the new tarsi canal implants has been observed. This is just an observation and further studies must be carried on to confirm this assumption (**Figs. 1–19**).

On the other hand, the calcaneo-stop procedure is a less expensive surgery compared with any of the other implants, and the authors have observed similar good results in terms of function and pain improvement. In the authors' opinion, tarsal canal implants produce better cosmetic correction compared with the calcaneo-stop technique in selected patients. This is another issue that needs further investigation for more consistent conclusions.

The authors have also observed better cosmetic correction with tarsi canal implants compared with sinus tarsi or calcaneo-stop procedures (**Figs. 20–25**).

BIOMECHANICS

Pisani[20] described the so-called coxa pedis comparing the hip with the talonavicular joint. Pisani also described the concept of a "glenopathy," in which the triplanar flat-foot deformity involves an insufficiency of the deltoid and spring ligaments. This is much closer to the way posterior tibial tendon dysfunction is currently believed consequence of insufficient medial ankle and foot structures. In this aspect the pediatric and the flexible flatfoot deformity in the adult are similar.

Table 1 Classification of arthroeresis procedures	
Classification	**Calcaneo Stop Technique**

A. Sinus tarsi implants
  1. Self-locking wedges
  2. Axis-altering implants
  3. Impact-blocking devices
	Figs. 1–19

B. Calcaneo stop
  1. Calcaneus
  2. Talus
	Figs. 20–25

C. Tarsi canal implants	Figs. 26–34

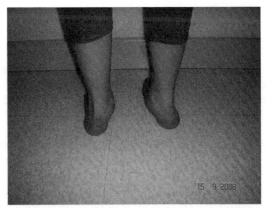

Fig. 1. Preoperative picture of flatfoot—frontal view after calcaneo-stop correction.

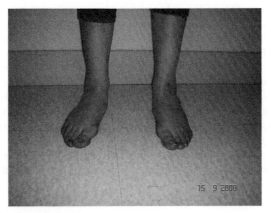

Fig. 2. Preoperative frontal picture.

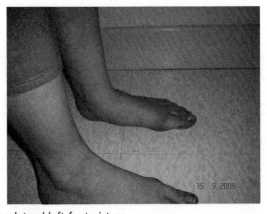

Fig. 3. Preoperative lateral left foot picture.

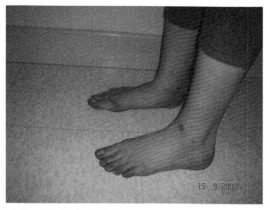

Fig. 4. Preoperative lateral right foot picture.

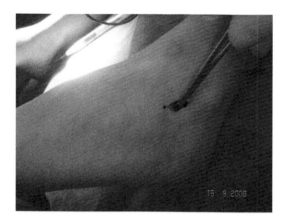

Fig. 5. Incision.

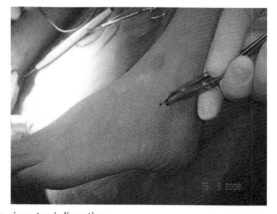

Fig. 6. Technique: sinus tarsi dissection.

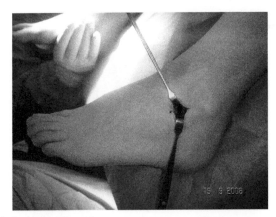

Fig. 7. Sinus tarsi view after dissection.

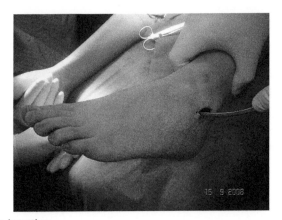

Fig. 8. Lever arm insertion.

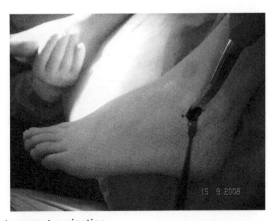

Fig. 9. Lever arm to correct supination.

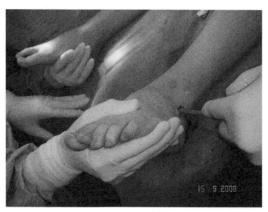

Fig. 10. Lever arm correction.

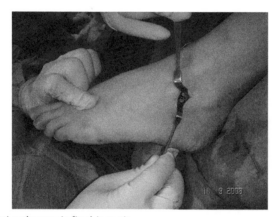

Fig. 11. Sinus tarsi arthrorrosis final insertion.

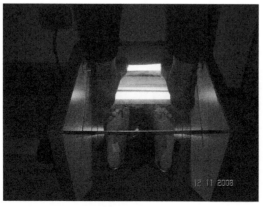

Fig. 12. Sinus tarsi arthrorrosis postoperative day 1.

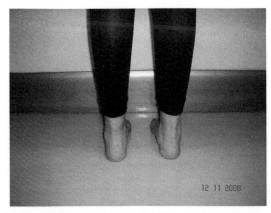

Fig. 13. Sinus tarsi arthrorrosis postoperative day 2.

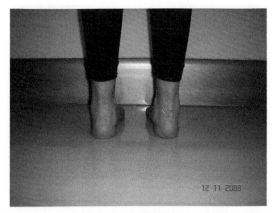

Fig. 14. Sinus tarsi arthrorrosis postoperative day 3.

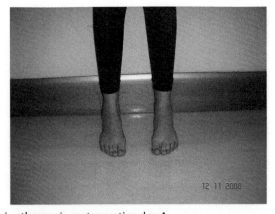

Fig. 15. Sinus tarsi arthrorrosis postoperative day 4.

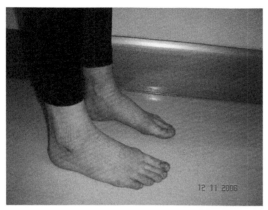

Fig. 16. Sinus tarsi arthrorrosis postoperative day 5.

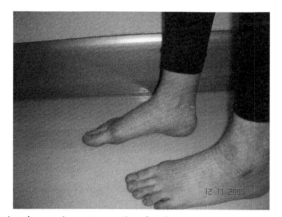

Fig. 17. Sinus tarsi arthrorrosis postoperative day 6.

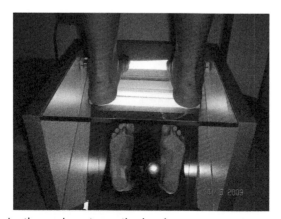

Fig. 18. Sinus tarsi arthrorrosis postoperative in mirror.

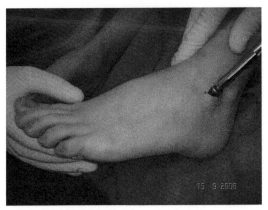

Fig. 19. Sinus tarsi arthrorrosis trial component.

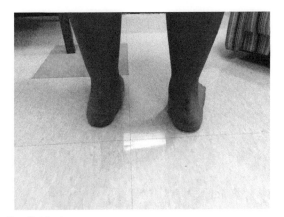

Fig. 20. Preoperative flatfoot.

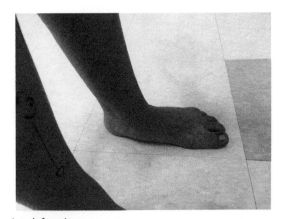

Fig. 21. Preoperative deformity.

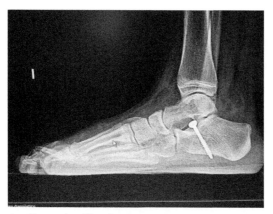

Fig. 22. Lateral foot radiograph with calcaneo stop.

Although the foot is not a single bone, it is useful to apply reconstruction principles to flatfoot deformity to understand it better. Classically, the deformity apex is located at the talonavicular joint, as discussed in the pediatric literature.[21] Regarding the foot divided in columns, the medial column is represented by the talus and first metatarsal and commences to deviate from the lateral column shaped by the calcaneus and lateral tarsal bones. The apex of the deformity is located at the subtalar joint.[22,23] This is the biomechanical reason why the arthroereisis procedure

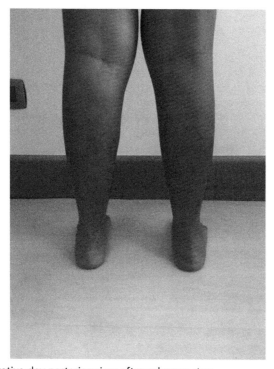

Fig. 23. Postoperative day posterior view after calcaneo stop.

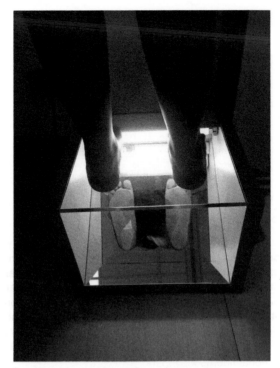

Fig. 24. Postoperative day arch correction after calcaeno stop.

is so efficient, because it acts at the apex of the deformity in a constrained structure.[18]

From a neuropropioceptive point of view, it is interesting to consider Pisani's observation of contralateral side deformity correction in patients operated on 1 side. This is supported by a recent description of the mirror cortical neuron as well as the rich concentration of mechanoreceptors in the subtalar joint.[24] This hypothesis might explain why a correction persists after implant removal. Further investigation is needed to fully understand how exactly arthroereisis works.

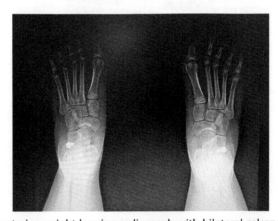

Fig. 25. Anteroposterior weight-bearing radiograph with bilateral calcaneo stop.

INDICATIONS

Most investigators agree that in cases of failure of conservative treatment, surgery can be considered. Because arthroereisis is an easy procedure with low risks and complications, a stretched or easy indication should be taken into consideration when compared with osteotomies and arthrodesis. Although it can also be used in adults, the majority of literature recommends its use between the ages of 8 years and 14 years.[25]

Viladot noted that, when performed in too young individuals, a tendency of cavovarus was seen. In addition, Roth[25] described more failures after arthroereisis when used later than age of 14 years.

These observation and recommendations, however, are lacking good level of evidence.

For an adult population, the technique is used as complementary procedure in conjunction with osteotomies and soft tissue reconstruction. Medial soft tissue reconstruction can benefit from this extra protection provided by the arthroereisis.

There is no consensus related to what kind of arthoerereisis should be indicated. Sinus tarsi and tarsi canal implants are more expensive than calcaneo-stop techniques. When comparing sinus tarsi with tarsal canal implants, it seems that the ones inserted into the canal have lower extrusion rates. Unfortunately, there is no level 1study in the literature available to prove which is best (**Figs. 26–35**).

A recent survey involved 1818 American Orthopaedic Foot and Ankle Society members, US and non-US surgeons. Of those, 404 responded. As a result, an increasing number of implants in the market have been found (>30). Non-US surgeons are still using the procedure in 53% whereas US surgeons are still using it in 24%. The rates of surgeons who have used the technique and kept on using it are higher in the rest of the world than in the US, as follows (have used it/are still using it):

Africa (100%/100%)
Australia (88%/81%)
Asia (68%/55%)
South America (67%/47%)
Europe 55%/45%
United States (41%/25%)[26]

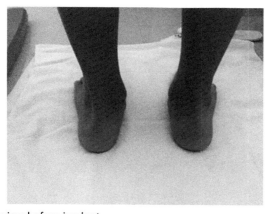

Fig. 26. Posterior view before implant.

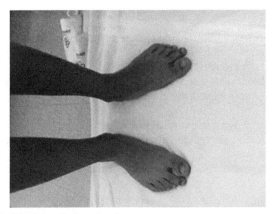

Fig. 27. Frontal flatfoot view before implant.

The authors' personal indication focuses on patients at an age between 10 years and 15 years old and who suffer from symptomatic but flexible flatfeet. All the patients should have undergone an adequate conservative treatment, which finally failed. The authors also consider this technique for adults with flatfeet in whom an extra protection of the reconstructed medial structures is found necessary. The most important indication for this technique in adults is that during surgery it becomes apparent that the correction with or without osteotomy is insufficient. Therefore, the implant is considered an adjunct to promote better control and correction.

SURGICAL TECHNIQUE

Independent of chosen type of implant or technique, most investigators perform a 2-cm incision directly over the sinus tarsi. The technique varies a little bit among all different types of implants available in the literature, but usually it does not take more than 20 minutes to accomplish the procedure (see **Figs. 6–11**).

REHABILITATION

The first reports recommended protected non–weight bearing in a cast, but recently most investigators have been shifting to a faster rehabilitation beginning weight

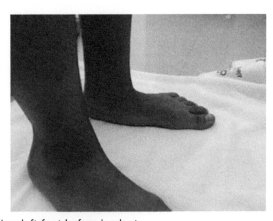

Fig. 28. Lateral view left foot before implant.

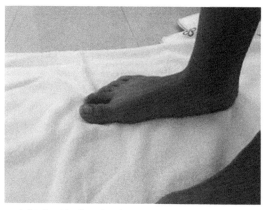

Fig. 29. Lateral view right foot before implant.

bearing in a removable boot as tolerated and progressive return to normal daily activities (Video 1).

Although there is no level 1 study reporting on the return to the sports level, a recent report investigated 49 consecutive patients. All patients were aged between 7 years and 14 years and treated surgically by means of an arthroereisis. The average follow-up was 5 years. Patients resumed their preoperative level of sporting activity within 1 year after surgery in terms of frequency, duration, and type.[27]

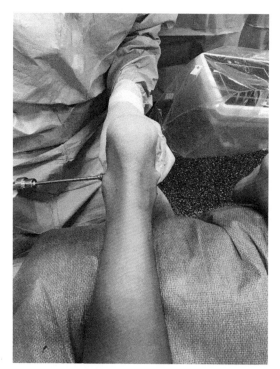

Fig. 30. Implant insertion from behind.

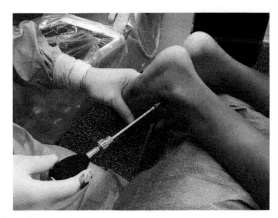

Fig. 31. Implant insertion.

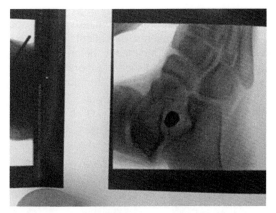

Fig. 32. Implant technique surgical radiograph.

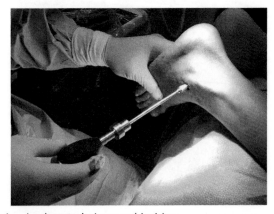

Fig. 33. Surgical view implant technique and incision.

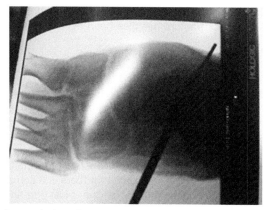

Fig. 34. X-ray implant technique intraoperative.

COMPLICATIONS

Arthroereisis is considered technically not demanding and quickly feasible. There are several complications, however, associated with this procedure. The most common is implant removal. A recent report by Saxena and colleagues[28] dealing with the use of arthroereisis in adult flatfoot deformity found an average hardware removal rate of 22.1% in 100 patients. Age was not a risk factor for implant removal but a size of more than 11 mm is indeed a risk factor for removal.

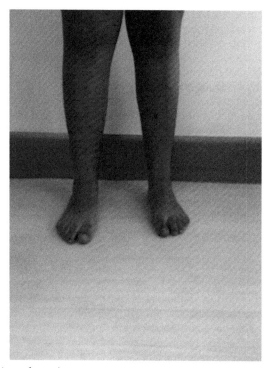

Fig. 35. Frontal view after calcaneo-stop correction.

Some specific and rare complications have been described, such as spontaneous subtalar fusion.[29] Talar neck fracture has also been described as well as sinus tarsi pain.[30]

DISCUSSION

The initial treatment of flexible flatfeet is conservative. When adequate treatment fails, however, and the foot remains symptomatic, surgical intervention should be considered. The classic surgical procedures for flatfoot reconstruction in adults and children include soft tissue procedures (ie, tendon transfers), osteotomies (lengthening and shifting), and arthrodesis. In acquired flatfeet cases, a large amount of literature has been published related to the mistakenly called "posterior tibial tendon dysfunction." Understanding of this condition now considers that there is a complete failure of the medial structures in which the posterior tibial tendon is just part and not the etiology of the problem. Although different combinations of procedures have been described, there is no consensus about the best treatment option in a specific case. What seems clear is that just medial soft tissue reconstruction is not enough and some bony procedure, which corrects the hindfoot and/or forefoot alignment, must be added to have successful and reliable results, the most frequent a calcaneal varizating osteotomy. Because most bony procedures involve a major foot surgery, the option of a simple, quick procedure sounds appealing.

In adolescents, in particular flexible flatfeet cases, an arthroereisis procedure maybe particularly useful between 8 years and 14 years of age but only when the children remain in pain after conservative treatment. Due to the successful rate of the arthroereisis procedure combined with low risk and complication rates, it can be considered in this particular kind of population.

The minimal invasiveness and short surgical time allow an early return to daily activities and do not burn any bridges for future treatment modalities. As discussed previously, the most striking complication is a potential hardware removal. The results seem to be left unaffected. There is still more evidence needed to get a better final conclusion regarding arthroereisis in younger individuals.

For the adult patient population, indications are even more confusing, but it seems reasonable to consider arthoereisis as a complement for other techniques to protect the medial soft tissue reconstructions or help improve corrective power associated with different kind of osteotomies.

The selection of type of arthroereisis seems to be surgeon preference. Most recent implants may increase the cost of treatment. Therefore, the cheaper calcaneo-stop procedures need to be kept in mind.

The low level of evidence available in the literature does not allow recommending arthroereisis in every case but seems robust enough to consider as a potential treatment option that could be added into the surgical armamentarium of orthopedic surgeons.

SUMMARY

One of the most common orthopedic problems found in an orthopedic practice is flatfoot deformity. Although this pathology is most commonly treated conservatively, there is still lack of consensus about the type of surgical treatment, which should be applied to patients who have not responded to nonoperative measures.

Isolated medial soft tissue reconstructions have not shown sufficient enough to correct a flatfoot deformity. In contrast, osteotomies and fusions are invasive procedures with their inherent risks for specific complications. Therefore, for certain specific patient populations, arthroereisis could be a valuable option, allowing quick surgical interventions with low rates of complications.

SUPPLEMENTARY DATA

Supplementary data related to this article can be found online at https://doi.org/10.1016/j.fcl.2018.04.010.

REFERENCES

1. Feciot CF. The etiology of developmental flatfoot. Clin Orthop 1972;85:7–10.
2. Staheli LT. Evaluation of planovalgus foot deformities with special reference to the natural history. J Am Podiatr Med Assoc 1987;77:2–6.
3. Giannini S, Ceccarelli F. The flexible flatfoot. Foot Ankle Clin 1998;4:573–92.
4. Lin YC, Kwon JY, Ghorbanhoseini M, et al. The hindfoot arch: what role does the imager play? Radiol Clin North Am 2016;54:951–68.
5. Root ML, Orien WP, Weed JH. Normal and abnormal function of the foot. Clin Biomech 1977;2:295–339.
6. Wenger DR, Leach J. Foot deformities in infant and children. Pediatr Clin North Am 1986;33:1411–27.
7. Viladot A. Surgical treatment of the child's flatfoot. Clin Orthop 1992;283:34–8.
8. Schon LC. Subtalar arthroereisis: a new exploration of an old concept. Foot Ankle Clin 2007;12:329–39.
9. Giannini S, Cadossi M, Mazzotti A, et al. Bioabsorbable calcaneo-stop implant for the treatment of flexible flatfoot: a retrospective cohort study at a minimum follow-up of 4 years. J Foot Ankle Surg 2017;56:776–82.
10. Needleman RL. Current topic review: subtalar arthroereisis for correction of flexible flatfoot. Foot Ankle Int 2005;26:336–46.
11. Zaret DI, Myerson MS. Arthroereisis of the subtalar joint. Foot Ankle Clin 2003; 8(3):605–17.
12. Grice DS. An extra-articular arthrodesis of the subastragalar joint for correction of paralytic flat feet in children. J Bone Joint Surg Am 1952;34:927–40.
13. Haraldsson S. Operative treatment of pes planovalgus staticus juvenilis. Acta Orthop Scand 1962;32:492–8.
14. Lelievre J. The valgus foot: current concepts and correction. Clin Orthop 1970;70: 43–55.
15. Gross RH. A clinical study of the Batchelor subtalar arthrodesis. J Bone Joint Surg Am 1976;58-A:343–9.
16. Subotnick S. The subtalar joint lateral extra-articular arthroereisis: a follow-up report. J Am Podiatry Assoc 1977;32:27–33.
17. Alvarez R. Calcaneo stop. Tecnica personal para el tratamiento quirurgico del pie plano-valgo del nino y adolescente joven. In: Epeldelgui T, editor. Pie plano y anomalias del antepie. Madrid (Spain): Madrid Vicente; 1995. p. 174–7 [in Spanish].
18. Usuelli FG, Montrasio UA. The calcaneo-stop procedure. Foot Ankle Clin N Am 2012;17:183–94.
19. Vogler HW. STJ blocking operation for pathologic pronation syndrome. In: McGlamry ED, editor. Comprehensive textbook of foot surgery. Baltimore (MD): Williams & Wilkins; 1987. p. 466–82.
20. Pisani G. Peritalar destabilization syndrome (adult flatfoot with degenerative glenopathy). Foot Ankle Surg 2010;16:183–8.

21. Moooa V. Flexible flatfoot in children and adolescents. J Child Orthop 2010;4: 107–21.
22. Cornwall MW, McPoil TG. Three-dimensionalmovementofthefootduringthestance phase of walking. J Am Podiatr Med Assoc 1999;89:56.
23. Kirby KA. Biomechanics of the normal and abnormal foot. J Am Podiatr Med Assoc 2000;90:30.
24. Molenberghs P, Hayward L, Mattingley JB, et al. Activation patterns during action observation are modulated by context in mirror system areas. Neuroimage 2012; 59(1):608–15.
25. Roth S, Sestan B, Tudor A, et al. Minimali nvasive calcaneo-stop method for idiopathic flexible per planovalgus in children. Foot Ankle Int 2007;28(9):991–5.
26. Shah NS, Needleman RL, Bokhari O, et al. 2013 Subtalar Arthroereisis Survey The Current Practice Patterns of Members of the AOFAS. Foot and ankle Specialist 2015;8(3):180–5.
27. Martinelli N, Bianchi A, Martinkevich P, et al. Return to sport activities after subtalar arthroereisis for correction of pediatric flexible flatfoot. J Pediatr Orthop B 2017;27(1):82–7.
28. Saxena A, Via AG, Maffulli N, et al. Subtalar arthroereisis implant removal in adults: a prospective study of 100 patients. J Foot Ankle Surg 2016;55(3):500–3.
29. Lui TH. Spontaneous subtalar fusion: an irreversible complication of subtalar arthroereisis. J Foot Ankle Surg 2014;53(5):652–6.
30. Kumar V, Clough TM. Talar neck fracture—A rare but important complication following subtalar arthroereisis*. Foot (Edinb) 2014;24:169–71.

Coalitions of the Tarsal Bones

Georg Klammer, MD[a],*, Norman Espinosa, MD[a], Lukas Daniel Iselin, MD[b]

KEYWORDS

- Tarsal coalition • Talocalcaneal • Calcaneonavicular • Management • Resection
- Fusion

KEY POINTS

- Tarsal coalitions develop due to failure of mesenchymal separation of tarsal bones.
- Most commonly coalitions are calcaneonavicular or talocalcaneal.
- Subtalar stiffness results in pathologic kinematics with increased risk of ankle sprains, most often planovalgus foot deformity and progressive joint degeneration.
- Resection of the coalition yields good results; tissue interposition may reduce the risk of reossification, and concomitant deformity should be addressed.
- The primary trigger to joint fusion is joint degeneration.

INTRODUCTION

Tarsal coalitions can present as osseous (synostosis), fibrous (syndesmosis), or cartilaginous (synchondrosis) connections between the tarsal bones, most commonly primary due to failure of mesenchymal separation.[1,2] Most coalitions found are calcaneonavicular and talocalcaneal; however, pretty much any 2 adjacent bones of the foot may be fused (**Fig. 1**). Any combination of coalitions can be found and even total coalitions[3] were described.

HISTORICAL PERSPECTIVE AND INCIDENCE

The entire historical perspective is summarized in **Table 1**. Clinical series estimate the incidence of tarsal coalitions about 1% to 6%; however, because they are often asymptomatic or undiagnosed the real incidence certainly might be higher.[2,4–7] Better accuracy may be obtained using cadaver series reporting rates of 12.7% to 13% in

Disclosure: None.
[a] Foot and Ankle Surgery, FussInstitut Zurich, Kappelistrasse 7, Zurich 8002, Switzerland; [b] Foot and Ankle Surgery, Department of Orthopaedic Surgery and Traumatology, Spitalstrasse 16, Kantonsspital Lucerne, Lucerne 6000, Switzerland
* Corresponding author.
E-mail address: klammer@fussinstitut.ch

Foot Ankle Clin N Am 23 (2018) 435–449
https://doi.org/10.1016/j.fcl.2018.04.011
1083-7515/18/© 2018 Elsevier Inc. All rights reserved.

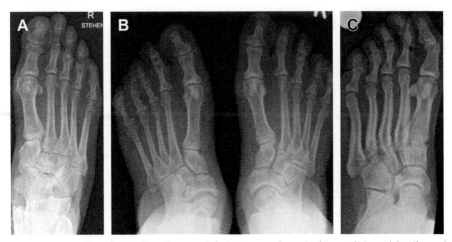

Fig. 1. Rare types of tarsal coalitions. (*A*) Osseous talonavicular coalition. (*B*) Bilateral osseous calcaneonavicular coalitions. (*C*) Fibrous naviculocuboidal coalition.

series of more than 100 dissected specimen.[8,9] MRI series on 574 consecutive patients revealed a similar rate of 11.5%.[5]

The most common found type is the calcaneonavicular coalition (53%–73%).[9,10] Together with the talocalcaneal coalition it accounts for greater than 90% of all tarsal coalitions[9]; 2.6% are either talonavicular or calcaneocuboid and the remaining distribute to various other connections of adjacent joints.[2,10]

Occurrence is bilateral in 50% to 68% overall,[2,4,10–12] calcaneonavicular in 40% to 60%, and talocalcaneal in 40% to 68%.[10,13] Coalitions distribute equally between the sexes or a male preponderance of up to 4:1 is found; however geographic variations may exist[2,13,14] (see **Table 1**).

CAUSE

Most coalitions are congenital. Leboucq in 1890 was the first to propose a failure of segmentation of primitive mesenchyme.[24] This is generally accepted since Harris found mesenchymal coalitions in fetal cadavers. However, today an autosomal dominant inherited pattern with a high penetrance is assumed.[11,13,25] Of patients with

Table 1 Historical perspective	
Buffon,[15] 1769	First description of tarsal coalition
Cruveilhier,[16] 1829	First anatomic description of calcaneonavicular coalition
Zuckerkandl,[17] 1877	First description of talocalcaneal coalition
Anderson,[18] 1880	First description of talonavicular coalition
Kirmisson,[19] 1898	First radiological description
Holland,[20] 1918	First description of calcaneocuboid coalition
Badgley,[21] 1927	First description of surgical resection of a calcaneonavicular bar, demonstrating regaining subtalar flexibility[22]
Waugh,[22] 1957	First description of cubonavicular coalition
Lusby,[23] 1959	First description of naviculocuneiform coalition

symptomatic tarsal coalitions, Leonard found asymptomatic coalitions in 39% of all and 76% of first-degree relatives. Coalition may be associated with other congenital malformations, for example, fibular hemimelia, symphalangism, Apert and Nievergelt-Pearlman syndromes, or proximal femoral deficiency.[11,26]

Rarely tarsal coalitions are secondary due to infection, arthritis, neoplasia, or trauma.[2]

PATHOPHYSIOLOGY

During the swing phase of gait the subtalar joint complex is positioned in a flexible valgus to accommodate for ground contact. During stance phase it changes into a rigid varus to allow effective translation of muscle force into body motion. External tibia rotation is compensated by subtalar internal rotation. If the coalition locks the subtalar joint motion, the gliding of the navicular and cuboid at the end of dorsiflexion is stopped and as a consequence the midtarsal joints need to compensate. The foot becomes flattened and the longitudinal arch is lost. This leads to adaptive shortening of the peroneal tendons and reactive spasm. Therefore, the term peroneal spastic flatfoot was coined to this pathology. Abnormal muscle activity of the peroneus longus has been shown electromyographically in various types of coalitions.[27] Altered subtalar kinematic eventually leads to posterior facet and midtarsal joint degeneration. At the Chopart joint a hingelike motion with repetitive navicular dorsal override develops the talar beaking due to capsular traction.[2,9,12,13,28,29]

Pain is thought to occur as ligament strains, sinus tarsi syndrome, and secondary joint degenerations.[30] Fibrocartilaginous coalitions are free of nerve fibers and pain likely results of repetitive microfractures and consequent remodeling through activation of periosteal nerve fibers.[31] When secondary joint degeneration develops, the source of pain sounds quite logic.[9]

Resection of the coalition attempts to restore normalized subtalar kinematics with minimized stress on the subtalar and adjacent joints. Although passive range of motion might be improved, Hetsroni and colleagues found similar severe restriction of kinematics in the pre- and postoperative analysis during walking.[32] Therefore, the effects of surgery may not be efficient enough regarding the functional result.

Ankle dorsiflexion in patients with tarsal coalition is reduced, tension on the Achilles tendon increased, and thus plantar pressures at the midfoot while a decrease is noted at the fifth metatarsal.[27] This explains the development of the pes planovalgus with midfoot breakdown and a pronation of the forefoot. These changes of plantar pressure persist after resection of the coalition and might imply the necessity of additional procedures to correct and balance the deformity.[27,33]

CLINICAL PRESENTATION

In adolescents who complain about foot pain tarsal coalition should always be kept in mind.[34] Timing of onset of symptoms is thought to correspond with the time of ossification and increasing stiffness of the foot.[10,35,36] In calcaneonavicular coalitions this typically occurs at age 8 to 12 years, whereas in talocalcaneal coalitions they ossify later (12–16 years).[37] Diffuse pain that exacerbates during activity is the main symptom and can be triggered by a minor trauma.[38] As a consequence patients start to modify and restrict their activity. Difficulty walking on uneven ground and repetitive ankle sprains should alert the clinician to consider coalition and assess subtalar motion meticulously.

The examination of gait may reveal a decreased stance phase due to pain. Typically the foot is in a planovalgus deformity with the forefoot hold in abduction. Normal and rarely rigid cavovarus may also occur in those patients.[12,39,40] Impaired subtalar motion is most pronounced in the middle facet talocalcaneal coalitions and is best assessed with the single-heel rise test showing a lack of hindfoot varisation or by letting the patient walk on the lateral border of the foot provoking discomfort.[2] The amount of restriction of the subtalar motion is variable and in up to 17% it might be normal.[40,41] Calcaneonavicular coalition usually expresses pain and tenderness at the sinus tarsi and over the peroneal tendons. In addition, a positive Silfverskjöld-Test revealing shortened calf muscles can be found. In talocalcaneal coalitions pain is located over the prominent sustentaculum tali and with increasing subtalar joint degeneration over the joint line medially and laterally. Rarely the protruding bone at the coalition leads to compression of the tibial nerve and thus symptoms of a tarsal tunnel syndrome.[42,43]

Subtalar motion should be assessed bilaterally while being aware of the frequent bilaterality of coalitions.

IMAGING

In 1921 Slomann was first to describe the identification of a calcaneonavicular coalition on plain radiograph.[44] For calcaneonavicular coalitions the 45° oblique view has a sensitivity of 90% to 100%. Talocalcaneal coalitions are more likely to be missed due to superimposed bony structures and their oblique orientation.[44,45] Fibrocartilaginous coalitions are identified by a decreased bony gap bordered by irregular sclerotic margins. Standard examination consists of weight-bearing ankle anteroposterior and dorsoplantar, oblique, and lateral views of the foot. Besides the typical radiological signs summarized in **Table 2**, hindfoot alignment can be assessed by using standardized angle measurements. Additional radiographs for hindfoot alignment such as the Saltzman or long-axial view may be obtained. Furthermore, alternative reasons for a rigid flatfoot deformity such as an accessory talar facet may be recognized[4,46] (**Figs. 2** and **3**).

Specific views allowing identification of talocalcaneal coalitions have been described, however, with increasing availability of computed tomography (CT) and MRI lost significance in daily practice.[53] CT was the standard imaging technique for the identification of tarsal coalitions; however, in 100 dissected feet Solomon and colleagues found 9 talocalcaneal or calcaneonavicular coalitions (all nonosseous) of which prior CT only identified 55% correctly. Furthermore, 4 suspected coalitions on CT could not be confirmed by anatomic dissection.[9] Diagnostic superiority of MRI in the diagnosis of coalitions was also shown by Guignand and colleagues[54,55] in a study of 19 patients with surgically proven calcaneonavicular coalitions where in contrast to MRI, CT had failed to identify 4 cases. The availability of MRI increased in the last 2 decades, whereas the cost commenced to decrease. Furthermore, radiation exposure for younger individuals is omitted. Thus MRI has become a golden standard in the assessment of coalitions. Sagittal and axial slices are best to appreciate calcaneonavicular, coronal slices for talocalcaneal coalitions. In bony coalitions medullary signal is found in continuation; in fibrocartilaginous types inflammatory signs of the bone margins and the surrounding soft tissues are observed. For surgical planning the spatial orientation of the coalition is studied and the amount of joint degeneration assessed.

Single photon emission computed tomography–CT scan allows locating szintigraphic activity with good spatial resolution on the superimposed CT slices (**Fig. 4**). Isolated activity at the site of coalition may help to identify it as source of complaints of the patient and concomitant activity within the joints in the decision between resection of the coalition or joint fusion when surgery is planned.

Table 2
Radiological signs of calcaneonavicular and talocalcaneal coalitions

Calcaneonavicular Coalition (see **Fig. 2**)

Bony bar sign[47]	Sensitivity 73%, specificity 100%
Anteater nose sign[47]	Elongated anterior calcaneal process in the lateral or oblique X-ray views Sensitivity 72%, specificity 94%[48]
Reversed anteater sign[47,49]	Elongated lateral navicular beyond the talar head in the oblique or dorsoplantar X-ray view Sensitivity 18%–50%, specificity 100%[48]
Talar beaking[45]	Capsular traction spur on the dorsal talar neck Sensitivity 49%, specificity 91%
Hypoplasia of the lateral talar head[2]	Best identified on the oblique X-ray view

Talocalcaneal Coalition (see **Fig. 3**)

C-Sign[50]	Circular confluence of talar dome and inferior margin of the sustentaculum on lateral views. May be positive in flatfoot deformity without coalition[51] Sensitivity 88%, specificity 87%[47]
Talar beaking[29,45]	Capsular traction spur on the dorsal talar neck (more common in talocalcaneal than calcaneonavicular coalitions) Sensitivity 48%, specificity 91%
Absent middle facet sign[52]	Absence of the middle facet in a true lateral view (allowing exclusion of the diagnosis if negative) Sensitivity 100%, specificity 42%
Short talar neck	Best identified on dorsoplantar or lateral radiograph
Drunken Waiter sign[2,37]	Enlarged dysmorphic sustentaculum holds an upturned joint line such as the hand of a drunken waiter holding the tray. Convex joint line shape instead of flat Sensitivity 82%, specificity 70%[47]

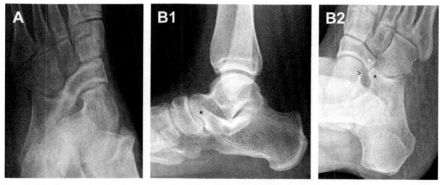

Fig. 2. Radiograph of calcaneonavicular coalition. (*A*) Synostosis: bony bar sign (oblique view). (*B1, B2*) Fibrous coalition (lateral and oblique views): Anteater sign (*black asterisk*), reversed anteater sign (*white asterisk*), hypoplasia of the lateral talar head (>).

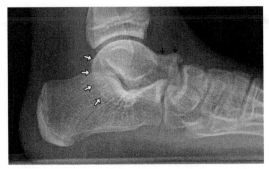

Fig. 3. Talocalcaneal coalition (lateral view). C-sign (*white arrows*) and talar beaking with short talar neck (*black arrows*).

NATURAL HISTORY

The fact that most coalitions remain asymptomatic through entire life is reflected by the difference between the incidences of clinical and cadaver or advanced imaging studies. Calcaneonavicular coalitions are less likely to progress into secondary joint degeneration and assumable because subtalar motion is less restricted.[9]

CONSERVATIVE TREATMENT

The first-line treatment consists of nonoperative treatment strategies. Activity modifications, antiinflammatory measures including nonsteroidal antirheumatics or corticoid injections and functional orthotics can be applied.[56] Physical therapy is used to address any peroneal and calf muscle tightness.[30] If pain relief is insufficient cast immobilization in a neutral position for 3 to 6 weeks can be offered. After cast removal 30% of patients may remain pain free but the response rate is worse for calcaneonavicular coalition when compared with the talocalcaneal coalitions.[57] Symptoms are less likely to resolve in older patients with long-standing symptoms or when signs of joint degeneration are present.[2,36,41,49,58] Remember that resection of calcaneonavicular coalition yield better results in younger patients (**Fig. 4**).

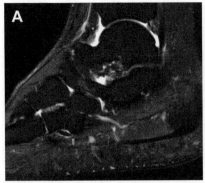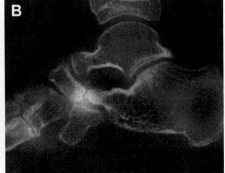

Fig. 4. Fibrous calcaneonavicular coalition demonstrating signs of inflammation (same patient as in **Fig. 2**B). (*A*) Sagittal MRI T2 weighted image. (*B*) Sagittal SPECT-CT image.

SURGICAL RESECTION OF THE COALITION
Resection of Calcaneonavicular Coalition

Failed conservative treatment may warrant surgical treatment.

The patient is positioned supine or in the lateral decubitus position. The investigators prefer Ollier approach over the sinus tarsi. Once the inferior extensor retinaculum is divided the surgeon advances to the coalition reflecting the muscle belly of the short toe extensor from its insertion on the calcaneus. Preventing to open the talonavicular joint capsule protects its cartilage and later subluxation. A bone block of at least 1 cm thickness is resected verifying sufficient removal medially, highlighting the importance of exact preoperative planning of the coalitions' spatial orientation on CT (or MRI) slices.[59] Swensen describes 2 lines helping to establish the margins of adequate resection: on the navicular side it is the extension of the lateral border of the talar neck and on the calcaneal side the medial border of the cuboid.[34]

In order to prevent any recurrence of ossification tissue interposition (eg, extensor digitorum brevis, fat or use of bone wax, hemostatic agents, and silicon sheets were proposed) can be considered.[34,37,60]

No (autologous) tissue interposition: Mitchell reported on relief of symptoms in 68% patients after an average follow-up of 6 years. In addition, in 58% of patients 25° of subtalar inversion could be achieved. But in one-third of the patients there was a recurrence of the coalition.[61] Supporters of tissue interposition often argue with retrospective series by Moyes and colleagues who found 3 recurrent ossifications in 7 patients without tissue interposition, whereas in the remaining 10 cases with extensor digitorum brevis interposition no recurrence was seen. However, Fuson and colleagues[38] reviewed their results of 25 patients treated in a 10-year period. Only a bar resection has been performed and bone wax used to cover the bony surfaces. Twenty-one patients remained asymptomatic at the time of follow-up.

Interposition of the extensor digitorum brevis (EDB): By means of a suture placed into the reflected muscle origin and passed through the resected coalition to exit the skin on the medial side of the foot, the muscle is pulled through the area of resection.[34] Cohen reported pain relief in 11 of 13 feet after a follow-up averaging 36 months. However, a high rate of wound complications occurred.[62,63] With a similar follow-up time of 2 to 3 years Gonzalez and colleagues published good to excellent results in 77% of patients in a series of 75 feet.[64] Van Renterghem and De Ridder found 95% of 22 teenage patients satisfied after a mean follow-up of nearly 5 years.[65] However, in a cadaver study Mubarak showed that the EDB could only fill 64% of the resected coalition and pointed out that the uncovered anterior process of the calcaneus leaves a sensitive and cosmetically poor prominence.[66] This is supported by several studies reporting complications with EDB interposition.[38,63] Conversely Scott and colleagues[56] encountered only minor complications in 7 patients with EDB interposition and good outcomes after, on average, more than 4.5 years follow-up.

Fat pad interposition: A 2-cm fat pad is usually harvested at the gluteal crease and interposed into the resected coalition and covered by reposition of the EDB.[34] In a retrospective analysis by Mubarak and colleagues,[66] 87% of patients had returned to sports and 74% of patients had improved subtalar motion. Long-term results were reported in a retrospective series by Swiontkowski and colleagues[29]: 74% were completely and 18% largely pain free with 90% restoration of subtalar motion in 90% of the cases.

More recent publications propose endoscopic surgical techniques. Resection of the coalition is achieved using an arthroscopic burr. The calcaneocuboid and talonavicular joints are used as margins of resection. No tissue is interposed and as in the open procedure the amount of resection is checked fluoroscopically.[67,68] So far only few case reports mainly in the adolescent to young adult population show the feasibility of the technique. In terms of the American Orthopedic Foot and Ankle (AOFAS) Score increases from 23 to 58 to 82 to 100 points good results were achieved.[69–72]

Generally favorable results of 78% to 90% are reported in the literature regarding the resection of calcaneonavicular coalitions.[38,58,73,74] Patients are less likely to quit their sports activities when compared with patients treated conservatively.[75] Similar favorable results were reported by Khosbin and colleagues[76] in a long-term follow-up of 14.4 years. Contradicting earlier studies, outcomes were not inferior after resection of calcaneonavicular compared with talocalcaneal coalitions.[75,76] Patients with resections of fibrocartilaginous coalitions perform better than those with bony co-alitions.[49,64] Progressive ossification of the coalition with age occurs and is associated with advanced joint degeneration. Patients with younger age (<14–16 years) at resection may yield better results.[37,64] However the degree of joint degeneration is more important than patient age when resection of the coalition is considered.[38,41,49,56,77] A study by Cohen and colleagues[63] focused on the outcomes in an adult population: 10 of 12 patients (13 feet) with an average age of 33 years reported pain relief after an average of 36 months. This is interesting because 75% of patients had already signs of degenerative changes at the time of surgery. Khosbin found a low reoperation rate of 15% after 9.5 years.[76] Secondary fusion rates have been reported to range between 4.5% and 16.6%.[63,76]

Resection of Calcaneonavicular Coalition with Concomitant Flatfoot Reconstruction

Flatfoot deformity is a common finding in patients with coalitions. Although for talocalcaneal coalitions the number of studies on bar resection in combination with deformity correction is growing, the evidence for calcaneonavicular coalitions is sparse.[78] Quinn and colleagues[79] demonstrated successful restoration of radiological angles with calcaneonavicular bar resection and flatfoot correction; however clinical data of the outcome are not yet available. The authors agree with Gougoulias and colleagues[30] that resection of a coalition should be accompanied by deformity correction using a tailored approach of soft-tissue and osseous procedures in order to balance loads.

Calcaneonavicular Coalition and Concomitant Stress Fractures

Petrover and colleagues[80] evaluated anterior process calcaneus stress fractures and found in 60% an association with calcaneonavicular coalitions. It could be that subtalar rigidity increases the risk of nonunion and was reported by Taketomi.[81] Nilsson and Coetzee earlier decided for a conservative treatment in Marathon runner who successfully returned to full activity within 4 months.[82] Pearce and colleagues,[83] on the other hand, decided for resection of the coalition (without tissue interposition) and screw fixation of the fracture in a patient professionally active in contact sports and as well had perfect recovery at 6 months.

Associated navicular stress fracture has to the authors' knowledge only been described once and had healed after resection without screw fixation of the fracture.[84]

Resection of Talocalcaneal Coalition

The patient is placed supine. The authors use a medial approach to the tarsus, which is located over the sustentaculum tali. The flexor retinaculum is released and the tendons of the tarsal tunnel are identified. The posterior tibial tendon is retracted dorsally and the long flexor posteriorly. The dorsal tendon sheath can be incised and the coalition is reached. By means of a scalpel the cartilaginous interface is identified. The coalition is resected with a 1 cm osteotome to free the joint completely. A bone block of at least 1 cm thickness is resected. Bone wax is placed on the bony surfaces. In order to confirm the accuracy of the resection, the range of motion at the hindfoot is tested and the posterior facet is visualized. If the mobility is not satisfying any possible capsular adhesions have to be resected. Autologous fat graft is harvested from the gluteal crease on the ipsilateral leg or a local subcutaneous fat pedicle may be used for interposition.[85–87] The graft is placed into the resected area and secured in place. The deep tendon sheath is now closed completely.

Assessment of the posterior facet through the open approach can be difficult, thus arthroscopic techniques have gained popularity in the past 5 years.[67] Knörr and colleagues[88] showed in their case review of 15 children promising results. Nevertheless this approach should remain in the hands of surgeons who are experienced with endoscopy.

As for calcaneonavicular coalitions, resection most commonly is advised usually with interposition of a fat pad[85] or use of bone wax. Wilde and colleagues[89] described in a series of 17 adolescent patients worse outcomes in patients with osseous coalitions of more than 50% and associated hindfoot valgus of more than 16% due to impingement of the lateral talar process on the calcaneus. However, later studies found quite favorable results in patients suffering from more extensive coalitions with higher degrees of hindfoot valgus.[90,91] In a retrospective review by Gantsoudes a series of 49 feet has been treated by means of open resection of the coalition and fat pad interposition. The average follow-up was 42.6 months. Of all patients 85% showed an excellent result with an average AOFAS score of 90/100. Notably 34% of patients underwent subsequent surgery to correct the alignment of the foot.[92]

Resection of a Talocalcaneal Coalition with Concomitant Flatfoot Reconstruction

As discussed earlier isolated resection of a talocalcaneal coalition tends to fail in case of associated flatfoot deformity due to the related functional deficit. Mosca and Bevan[93] and Masquijno and colleagues[94] reported on successful results after flatfoot correction using a calcaneal lengthening osteotomy in patients with resected talocalcaneal coalitions (<50%) and those in which coalitions of less than 50% were left unresected. Combining resection of coalitions less than 50% with medial displacement osteotomies, El-Shazly and colleagues[95] reported of significant improvements of pain VAS and AOFAS scores in a larger series of 30 resected feet. Even though most investigators respect the 50% limit of osseous coalition when indicating resection,[89] it has to be noted that Khosbin demonstrated good results with resection in patients with talocalcaneal bars of more than 50% and more than 16% in those with hindfoot valgus.[96] The authors, therefore, favor according to Zhou the combination with a flatfoot reconstruction in a single-stage operation.[97]

Complications of Resection

Possible complications of resection include wound healing impairment, infection, sural neuropathy, recurrent ossification or incomplete resection, subluxation of the talonavicular joint, and progressive joint degeneration. Endoscopic techniques have a longer learning curve but possibly cause less local morbidity.[67]

Postoperative Management

Postoperatively usually a regimen of 3 weeks of non–weight-bearing in a short leg cast is recommended, starting progressive weight-bearing and subtalar range of motion exercises at 4 weeks.[34]

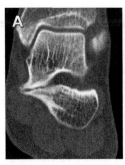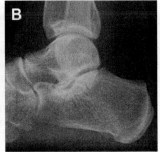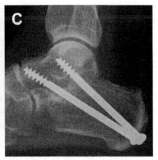

Fig. 5. Fibrous talocalcaneal coalition. (*A*) Preoperative coronary CT scan. (*B*) Preoperative lateral X-ray view. (*C*) Postoperative lateral X-ray view after successful joint fusion.

JOINT FUSION IN TARSAL COALITION

In case of multiple coalitions, failed primary resection and/or joint degeneration fusion is considered (**Fig. 5**). Fuson and colleagues[38] found that the level of pain was the determining factor to decide for joint fusion. Therefore, resection of coalitions should not be confined to adolescent patients. Good results have been shown not to depend on age as long as no joint degeneration has occurred.[63,98] The talar beak is caused by traction of the capsule and should not be misinterpreted as arthritic changes.[13] In a cohort study of 304 patients 5.3% had undergone joint fusion.[76]

The available studies on the outcomes of surgical treatment of tarsal coalitions are not sufficient to draw proper conclusions. Most studies are retrospective series without control groups, small study populations, and variable types of coalitions. In addition, measurements are of variable technique and often assessed using nonvalidated instruments.[40]

Subtalar joint fusion is a valuable solution for failed and symptomatic tarsal coalition surgeries. According to the underlying condition, the fusion has to be corrective to reduce mainly hindfoot valgus. Subtalar fusion can be achieved by an open or arthroscopically assisted procedure.

Double or triple arthrodesis is usually not aimed at in a juvenile population.[99]

SUMMARY

Tarsal coalitions are the result of impaired mesenchymal separation of the tarsal bones. The most common types include calcaneonavicular or talocalcaneal coalitions. They usually get first time symptomatic because of an ankle sprain. Subtalar stiffness results in pathologic kinematics with increased risk of ankle sprains, planovalgus foot deformity, and progressive joint degeneration.

Resection of the coalition yields good results. Tissue interposition may reduce the risk of reossification, and concomitant deformity should be addressed in the same surgical setting.

The primary trigger to joint fusion is marked joint degeneration.

REFERENCES

1. Upasani VV, Chambers RC, Mubarak SJ. Analysis of calcaneonavicular coalitions using multi-planar three-dimensional computed tomography. J Child Orthop 2008;2(4):301–7.
2. Zaw H, Calder JDF. Tarsal coalitions. Foot Ankle Clin 2010;15(2):349–64.

3. Reddy Mettu R, Koduru SK, Surath H, et al. Total bilateral tarsal coalition: a case report. J Foot Ankle Surg 2016;55(5):1035–7.

4. Lysack JT, Fenton PV. Variations in calcaneonavicular morphology demonstrated with radiography. Radiology 2004;230(2):493–7.

5. Nalaboff KM, Schweitzer ME. MRI of tarsal coalition: frequency, distribution, and innovative signs. Bull NYU Hosp Jt Dis 2008;66(1):14–21.

6. Pfitzner W. Beiträge zur Kenntnis des menschlichen Extremitätenskelets VI. Die Variationen im Aufbau des Fusskelets. In: Schwalbe G, editor. Morphologisches Arbeiten. Jena, Germany: Gustav Fischer; 1896. p. 245–527.

7. Wray JB, Herndon CN. Hereditary transmission of congenital coalition of the calcaneus to the navicular. JBJS 1963;45(2):365.

8. Rühli FJ, Solomon LB, Henneberg M. High prevalence of tarsal coalitions and tarsal joint variants in a recent cadaver sample and its possible significance. Clin Anat 2003;16(5):411–5.

9. Solomon LB, Rühli FJ, Taylor J, et al. A dissection and computer tomograph study of tarsal coalitions in 100 cadaver feet. J Orthop Res 2003;21(2):352–8.

10. Stormont DM, Peterson HA. The relative incidence of tarsal coalition. Clin Orthop 1983;181:28–36.

11. Leonard MA. The inheritance of tarsal coalition and its relationship to spastic flat foot. J Bone Joint Surg Br 1974;56B(3):520–6.

12. Mosier KM, Asher M. Tarsal coalitions and peroneal spastic flat foot. A review. J Bone Joint Surg Am 1984;66(7):976–84.

13. Vu L, Mehlman CT. Tarsal coalition. EMedicine spec orthop surg foot ankkle. Medscape 2016.

14. Conway JJ, Cowell HR. Tarsal coalition: clinical significance and roentgenographic demonstration. Radiology 1969;92(4):799–811.

15. Buffon GL. Compte de: Histoire Naturelle generale et particuliere. Paris: Imprimiere Royale; 1769.

16. Cruveilhier J. Anatomie pathologique du corps humian. J.B Bailliere 1829.

17. Zuckerkandl E. Über einen Fall von Synostose zwischen Talus und Calcaneus. Allg Wien Med Ztg 1877;22:293–4.

18. Anderson RJ. The presence of an astragalo-scaphoid bone in man. J Anat Physiol 1880;14(4):452–5.

19. Kirmisson E. Double pied bot varus par malformation osseuse primitive associe a des ankyloses congenitales des doigts et des orteils chez quatre membres d'une meme Famille. Rev Orthop 1898;9:392–8.

20. Holland CT. Two cases of rare deformity of feet and hands. Arch Radiol Electrother 1918;22:234–9.

21. Badgley C. Coalitions of the calcaneus and the navicular. Arch Surg 1927;15:75–88.

22. Waugh W. Partial cubo-navicular coalition as a cause of peroneal spastic flat foot. J Bone Jt Surg Br 1957;39:520–3.

23. Lusby HL. Naviculo-cuneiform synostosis. J Bone Joint Surg Br 1959;41–B(1):150.

24. Leboucq H. De la soudure congenitale de certains os du tarse. Bull Acad R Méd Belg 1890;4:103–12.

25. Mosca VS. Tarsal coalitions. 7th edition. Philadelphia: Lippincott Williams & Wilkins; 2014.

26. Grogan DP, Holt GR, Ogden JA. Talocalcaneal coalition in patients who have fibular hemimelia or proximal femoral focal deficiency. A comparison of the radiographic and pathological findings. J Bone Joint Surg Am 1994;76(9):1363–70.

27. Lyon R, Liu X-C, Cho S-J. Effects of tarsal coalition resection on dynamic plantar pressures and electromyography of lower extremity muscles. J Foot Ankle Surg 2005;44(4):252–8.
28. Nester CJ, Findlow AF, Bowker P, et al. Transverse plane motion at the ankle joint. Foot Ankle Int 2003;24(2):164–8.
29. Swiontkowski MF, Scranton PE, Hansen S. Tarsal coalitions: long-term results of surgical treatment. J Pediatr Orthop 1983;3(3):287–92.
30. Gougoulias N, O'Flaherty M, Sakellariou A. Taking out the tarsal coalition was easy: but now the foot is even flatter. What now? Foot Ankle Clin 2014;19(3): 555–68.
31. Kumai T, Takakura Y, Akiyama K, et al. Histopathological study of nonosseous tarsal coalition. Foot Ankle Int 1998;19(8):525–31.
32. Hetsroni I, Nyska M, Mann G, et al. Subtalar kinematics following resection of tarsal coalition. Foot Ankle Int 2008;29(11):1088–94.
33. Hetsroni I, Ayalon M, Mann G, et al. Walking and running plantar pressure analysis before and after resection of tarsal coalition. Foot Ankle Int 2007;28(5): 575–80.
34. Swensen SJ, Otsuka NY. Tarsal coalitions–calcaneonavicular coalitions. Foot Ankle Clin 2015;20(4):669–79.
35. Katayama T, Tanaka Y, Kadono K, et al. Talocalcaneal coalition: a case showing the ossification process. Foot Ankle Int 2005;26(6):490–3.
36. Lemley F, Berlet G, Hill K, et al. Current concepts review: tarsal coalition. Foot Ankle Int 2006;27(12):1163–9.
37. Cowell HR. Talocalcaneal coalition and new causes of peroneal spastic flatfoot. Clin Orthop 1972;85:16–22.
38. Fuson S, Barrett M. Resectional arthroplasty: treatment for calcaneonavicular coalition. J Foot Ankle Surg 1998;37(1):11–5.
39. Stuecker RD, Bennett JT. Tarsal coalition presenting as a pes cavo-varus deformity: report of three cases and review of the literature. Foot Ankle 1993;14(9): 540–4.
40. Thorpe SW, Wukich DK. Tarsal coalitions in the adult population: does treatment differ from the adolescent? Foot Ankle Clin 2012;17(2):195–204.
41. Varner KE, Michelson JD. Tarsal coalition in adults. Foot Ankle Int 2000;21(8): 669–72.
42. Lee MF, Chan PT, Chau LF, et al. Tarsal tunnel syndrome caused by talocalcaneal coalition. Clin Imaging 2002;26(2):140–3.
43. Yamamoto S, Tominaga Y, Yura S, et al. Tarsal tunnel syndrome with double causes (ganglion, tarsal coalition) evoked by ski boots. Case report. J Sports Med Phys Fitness 1995;35(2):143–5.
44. Slomann HC. On coaltion calcaneo-navicularis. J Orthop Surg 1921;3:586–602.
45. Newman JS, Newberg AH. Congenital tarsal coalition: multimodality evaluation with emphasis on CT and MR imaging. Radiographics 2000;20(2):321–32 [quiz: 526–7, 532].
46. Niki H, Aoki H, Hirano T, et al. Peroneal spastic flatfoot in adolescents with accessory talar facet impingement: a preliminary report. J Pediatr Orthop B 2015;24(4): 354–61.
47. Crim JR, Kjeldsberg KM. Radiographic diagnosis of tarsal coalition. AJR Am J Roentgenol 2004;182(2):323–8.
48. Lawrence DA, Rolen MF, Haims AH, et al. Tarsal coalitions: radiographic, CT, and MR imaging findings. HSS J 2014;10(2):153–66.
49. Jayakumar S, Cowell HR. Rigid flatfoot. Clin Orthop 1977;122:77–84.

50. Lateur LM, Van Hoe LR, Van Ghillewe KV, et al. Subtalar coalition: diagnosis with the C sign on lateral radiographs of the ankle. Radiology 1994;193(3):847–51.

51. Brown RR, Rosenberg ZS, Thornhill BA. The C sign: more specific for flatfoot deformity than subtalar coalition. Skeletal Radiol 2001;30(2):84–7.

52. Liu PT, Roberts CC, Chivers FS, et al. "Absent middle facet": a sign on unenhanced radiography of subtalar joint coalition. AJR Am J Roentgenol 2003; 181(6):1565–72.

53. Harris RI, Beath T. Etiology of peroneal spastic flat foot. J Bone Joint Surg Br 1948;30B(4):624–34.

54. el Hayek T, D'Ollone T, Rubio A, et al. A too-long anterior process of the calcaneus: a report of 31 operated cases. J Pediatr Orthop B 2009;18(4):163–6.

55. Guignand D, Journeau P, Mainard-Simard L, et al. Child calcaneonavicular coalitions: MRI diagnostic value in a 19-case series. Orthop Traumatol Surg Res 2011;97(1):67–72.

56. Scott AT, Tuten HR. Calcaneonavicular coalition resection with extensor digitorum brevis interposition in adults. Foot Ankle Int 2007;28(8):890–5.

57. Bohne WH. Tarsal coalition. Curr Opin Pediatr 2001;13(1):29–35.

58. Mosca VS. Flexible flatfoot and tarsal coaltions and pes planovalgus: clinical exam, imaging and surgical planning. Rosemont (IL): American Academy of Orthopaedic Surgeos; 1996.

59. Espinosa N, Dudda M, Andersen J, et al. Prediction of spatial orientation and morphology of calcaneonavicular coalitions. Foot Ankle Int 2008;29(2):205–12.

60. Krief E, Ferraz L, Appy-Fedida B, et al. Tarsal coalitions: preliminary results after operative excision and silicone sheet interposition in children. J Foot Ankle Surg 2016;55(6):1264–70.

61. Mitchell GP, Gibson JM. Excision of calcaneo-navicular bar for painful spasmodic flat foot. J Bone Joint Surg Br 1967;49(2):281–7.

62. Cohen AH, Laughner TE, Pupp GR. Calcaneonavicular bar resection. A retrospective review. J Am Podiatr Med Assoc 1993;83(1):10–7.

63. Cohen BE, Davis WH, Anderson RB. Success of calcaneonavicular coalition resection in the adult population. Foot Ankle Int 1996;17(9):569–72.

64. Gonzalez P, Kumar SJ. Calcaneonavicular coalition treated by resection and interposition of the extensor digitorum brevis muscle. J Bone Joint Surg Am 1990;72(1):71–7.

65. Van Renterghem D, De Ridder K. Resection of calcaneonavicular bar with interposition of extensor digitorum brevis. A questionnaire review. Acta Orthop Belg 2011;77(1):83–7.

66. Mubarak SJ, Patel PN, Upasani VV, et al. Calcaneonavicular coalition: treatment by excision and fat graft. J Pediatr Orthop 2009;29(5):418–26.

67. Bonasia DE, Phisitkul P, Amendola A. Endoscopic coalition resection. Foot Ankle Clin 2015;20(1):81–91.

68. Lui TH. Arthroscopic resection of the calcaneonavicular coalition or the "too long" anterior process of the calcaneus. Arthroscopy 2006;22(8):903.e1-4.

69. Bauer T, Golano P, Hardy P. Endoscopic resection of a calcaneonavicular coalition. Knee Surg Sports Traumatol Arthrosc 2010;18(5):669–72.

70. Knörr J, Accadbled F, Abid A, et al. Arthroscopic treatment of calcaneonavicular coalition in children. Orthop Traumatol Surg Res OTSR 2011;97(5):565–8.

71. Molano-Bernardino C, Bernardino CM, Golanó P, et al. Experimental model in cadavera of arthroscopic resection of calcaneonavicular coalition and its first in-vivo application: preliminary communication. J Pediatr Orthop Part B 2009;18(6): 347–53.

72. Singh AK, Parsons SW. Arthroscopic resection of calcaneonavicular coalition/ malunion via a modified sinus tarsi approach: an early case series. Foot Ankle Surg 2012;18(4):266–9.

73. O'Neill DB, Micheli LJ. Tarsal coalition. A followup of adolescent athletes. Am J Sports Med 1989;17(4):544–9.

74. Skwara A, Zounta V, Tibesku CO, et al. Plantar contact stress and gait analysis after resection of tarsal coalition. Acta Orthop Belg 2009;75(5):654–60.

75. Saxena A, Erickson S. Tarsal coalitions. Activity levels with and without surgery. J Am Podiatr Med Assoc 2003;93(4):259–63.

76. Khoshbin A, Bouchard M, Wasserstein D, et al. Reoperations after tarsal coalition resection: a population-based study. J Foot Ankle Surg 2015;54(3):306–10.

77. Davis WH. Tarsal coalition. In: Nunley JA, Pfeffer GB, Sanders RW, editors. Advanced reconstruction of the foot and ankle. Rosemoent (IL): AAOS; 2004. p. 133–6.

78. Cass AD, Camasta CA. A review of tarsal coalition and pes planovalgus: clinical examination, diagnostic imaging, and surgical planning. J Foot Ankle Surg 2010; 49(3):274–93.

79. Quinn EA, Peterson KS, Hyer CF. Calcaneonavicular coalition resection with pes planovalgus reconstruction. J Foot Ankle Surg 2016;55(3):578–82.

80. Petrover D, Schweitzer ME, Laredo JD. Anterior process calcaneal fractures: a systematic evaluation of associated conditions. Skeletal Radiol 2007;36(7): 627–32.

81. Taketomi S, Uchiyama E, Iwaso H. Stress fracture of the anterior process of the calcaneus: a case report. Foot Ankle Spec 2013;6(5):389–92.

82. Nilsson LJ, Coetzee JC. Stress fracture in the presence of a calcaneonavicular coalition: a case report. Foot Ankle Int 2006;27(5):373–4.

83. Pearce CJ, Zaw H, Calder JDF. Stress fracture of the anterior process of the calcaneus associated with a calcaneonavicular coalition: a case report. Foot Ankle Int 2011;32(1):85–8.

84. Tanaka Y, Takakura Y, Akiyama K, et al. Fracture of the tarsal navicular associated with calcaneonavicular coalition: a case report. Foot Ankle Int 1995;16(12): 800–2.

85. Murphy JS, Mubarak SJ. Talocalcaneal coalitions. Foot Ankle Clin 2015;20(4): 681–91.

86. Imajima Y, Takao M, Miyamoto W, et al. Mid-term outcome of talocalcaneal coalition treated with interposition of a pedicle fatty flap after resection. Foot Ankle Int 2012;33(3):226–30.

87. Miyamoto W, Takao M, Uchio Y, et al. Technique tip: interposition of the pedicle fatty flap after resection of the talocalcaneal coalition. Foot Ankle Int 2007; 28(12):1298–300.

88. Knörr J, Soldado F, Menendez ME, et al. Arthroscopic talocalcaneal coalition resection in children. Arthrosc J Arthrosc Relat Surg 2015;31(12):2417–23.

89. Wilde PH, Torode IP, Dickens DR, et al. Resection for symptomatic talocalcaneal coalition. J Bone Joint Surg Br 1994;76(5):797–801.

90. Luhmann SJ, Schoenecker PL. Symptomatic talocalcaneal coalition resection: indications and results. J Pediatr Orthop 1998;18(6):748–54.

91. McCormack TJ, Olney B, Asher M. Talocalcaneal coalition resection: a 10-year follow-up. J Pediatr Orthop 1997;17(1):13–5.

92. Gantsoudes GD, Roocroft JH, Mubarak SJ. Treatment of talocalcaneal coalitions. J Pediatr Orthop 2012;32(3):301–7.

93. Mosca VS, Bevan WP. Talocalcaneal tarsal coalitions and the calcaneal lengthening osteotomy: the role of deformity correction. J Bone Joint Surg Am 2012; 94(17):1584–94.

94. Masquijo J, Vazquez I, Allende V, et al. Surgical reconstruction for talocalcaneal coalitions with severe hindfoot valgus deformity. J Pediatr Orthop 2017;37(4): 293–7.

95. El Shazly O, Mokhtar M, Abdelatif N, et al. Coalition resection and medial displacement calcaneal osteotomy for treatment of symptomatic talocalcaneal coalition: functional and clinical outcome. Int Orthop 2014;38(12):2513–7.

96. Khoshbin A, Law PW, Caspi L, et al. Long-term functional outcomes of resected tarsal coalitions. Foot Ankle Int 2013;34(10):1370–5.

97. Zhou B, Tang K, Hardy M. Talocalcaneal coalition combined with flatfoot in children: diagnosis and treatment: a review. J Orthop Surg 2014;9:129.

98. Vincent KA. Tarsal coalition and painful flatfoot. J Am Acad Orthop Surg 1998; 6(5):274–81.

99. Beimers L, de Leeuw PAJ, van Dijk CN. A 3-portal approach for arthroscopic subtalar arthrodesis. Knee Surg Sports Traumatol Arthrosc 2009;17(7):830–4.

Medial Approach to the Subtalar Joint

James Widnall, MB ChB, MRCS, FRCS (Tr&Orth)[a],
Lyndon Mason, MB BCh, MRCS (Eng), FRCS (Tr&Orth)[b],
Andrew Molloy, MB ChB, MRCS (Ed), FRCS (Tr&Orth)[b],*

KEYWORDS

- Subtalar joint • Hind foot arthrodesis • Double fusion • Medial approach
- Triple fusion • Subtalar arthroscopy

KEY POINTS

- The medial subtalar joint approach uses a window between the superficial ligaments, the tibiocalcaneal and spring ligament, thus maintaining much of the medial stability the hindfoot, although the tibiospring ligament is sacrificed.
- Medial arthroscopic approaches to the subtalar joint have been described, although the evidence is sparse.
- The talonavicular joint is the key to hindfoot motion.
- Greater than 90% of the subtalar joint and talonavicular joint are accessible from the medial approach.

INTRODUCTION

Surgical access to the subtalar joint is required in a plethora of pathologic conditions of the hindfoot. The conventional lateral approach can give excellent access to subtalar joint; however, in hindfoot valgus deformities, there can be unacceptable risks of wound problems and incomplete deformity corrections.[1,2] The medial approach to the subtalar joint has been popularized by many investigators, especially in hindfoot arthrodesis procedures in tibialis posterior dysfunction.[1,3-6] The authors' aim is to review the medial approach to the subtalar joint.

ANATOMY OF MEDIAL APPROACH TO SUBTALAR JOINT

The subtalar joint can be divided into 2 parts, anterior and posterior. Anteriorly, the talar head is located on the anterior and middle facets of the calcaneus, forming

[a] Trauma and Orthopaedic Department, Aintree University Hospital, Lower Lane, Liverpool, L9 7AL, UK; [b] Trauma and Orthopaedic Department, Aintree University Hospital, Liverpool University, Liverpool, UK
* Corresponding author. 7 Croome Drive, West Kirby, Wirral CH48 8AD, UK.
E-mail address: andymolloy3@gmail.com

Foot Ankle Clin N Am 23 (2018) 451–460
https://doi.org/10.1016/j.fcl.2018.04.006
1083-7515/18/© 2018 Elsevier Inc. All rights reserved.

the acetabulum pedis with the posterior surface of the navicular bone.[7] Movement at the acetabulum pedis is coupled to the movement of the subtalar joint. The posterior facet is larger than the middle and the anterior facets and is separated from the other 2 facets by the interosseous calcaneal ligament.[8] The sustentaculum tali is formed by the middle calcaneal facet (dorsal surface) and provides a sliding surface for 3 tendons (plantar surface): the tibialis posterior, flexor hallucis longus, and flexor digitorum longus tendons.[7,8] Galli and colleagues[9] scrutinized the medial approach with regards to proximity of local anatomic structures of importance. They demonstrated, on cadaveric specimens, a mean distance from the middle facet subtalar joint to the flexor digitorum longus (5 mm), flexor hallucis longus (19 mm), and the neurovascular bundle (21 mm). The tibialis posterior tendon was found to be less than 2 mm away from the middle facet of the subtalar joint but is useful as a landmark and to aid retraction.

The medial ligaments to the hindfoot are wide, variable complex structures that extend from the medial malleolus to the navicular, talus, and calcaneum. Milner and Soames[10] observed in 40 cadaveric specimens, 6 different components of the deltoid ligament of the ankle: 4 superficial (tibiospring, tibionavicular, superficial posterior tibiotalar, and tibiocalcaneal ligament), of which only the tibiospring and the tibionavicular were constant. They also observed 2 deep components: a deep posterior tibiotalar ligament and a deep anterior tibiotalar ligament, of which only the posterior tibiotalar ligament was constant. Boss and Hintermann[11] found that tibiocalcaneal and tibiospring ligaments were the longest, and the tibiocalcaneal and posterior deep tibiotalar ligaments are the thickest of these ligaments. The deep deltoid ligaments are relatively protected during the medial approach to the subtalar joint due to their attachment to the medial talar body. The superficial ligaments are at greater risk. **Fig. 1** illustrates the superficial ligamentous structures of the medial hindfoot and their relative position as described by Boss and Hintermann.[11] The superficial ligaments are often inseparable and blend with one another. A window between the tibiocalcaneal and spring ligament is possible, thus maintaining much of stability provided by the superficial ligaments, although the tibiospring ligament is sacrificed.

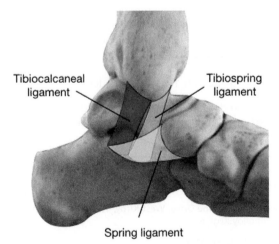

Tibiocalcaneal ligament

Tibiospring ligament

Spring ligament

Fig. 1. Skeleton of the medial hindfoot showing the origin and insertions of the superficial medial ligaments (tibiocalcaneal ligaments, tibiospring ligament, and spring ligament).

OPERATIVE TECHNIQUE FOR OPEN MEDIAL APPROACH TO THE SUBTALAR JOINT

The authors use a modification of the approach described by Jeng and colleagues[4]:

- The patient is placed supine on the operating table. In the authors' practice, a pneumatic thigh tourniquet is used.
- In cases of hindfoot valgus deformity, it is normal in the authors' practice to perform a medial head of gastrocnemius recession through a small posteromedial calf incision, 5 cm distal to the knee flexion crease.
- For the medial subtalar approach, the skin incision is made from just posterior to the medial malleolus to just distal to the navicular bone, parallel to and just above the tendon of tibialis posterior (**Fig. 2**).
- Careful dissection and cautery of the numerous venous plexuses is performed superficial to the tendon sheath of tibialis posterior. The tendon sheath is opened, and the tendon is inspected (**Fig. 3**). The posterior tibialis tendon is often tendinopathic, and the decision to excise the tendon may be taken. Without the posterior tibialis tendon in place, exposure of the medial aspect of the subtalar joint is easier; nevertheless, retaining the tendon still allows access to the joint.
- Identify the sustentaculum tali at the base of the posterior tibialis tendon sheath and use the superior aspect of the bony ridge to give access to the medial facet of the subtalar joint. Extensions can be made both anterior and posterior from this access point, with attempts to preserve the tibiocalcaneal ligament, which is posterior, and the spring ligaments, which are inferior. With the use of pin distractors or a lamina spreader between the talus and the calcaneus, access to the subtalar joint can be obtained (**Fig. 4**).
- The interosseous ligament can be transected to allow access to the anterior and posterior facets.
- If access to the talonavicular joint is required, a longitudinal incision can be made in the capsule of the talonavicular joint, exposing the head of the talus and the navicular bone (**Figs. 5** and **6**).

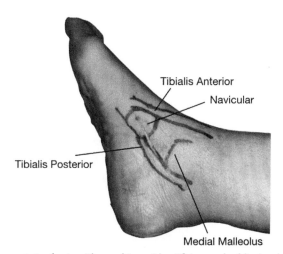

Tibialis Anterior

Navicular

Tibialis Posterior

Medial Malleolus

Fig. 2. Medial aspect to foot with markings identifying palpable landmarks, navicular, medial malleolus, tibialis anterior, and tibialis posterior tendons. Incision performed from posterior aspect of medial malleolus to navicular, superior to the course of the tibialis posterior tendon.

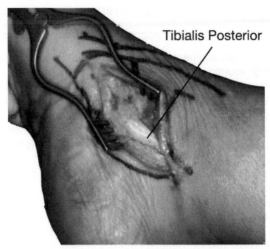

Fig. 3. The tibialis posterior tendon following the opening of the tibialis posterior tendon sheath.

- Because of the incision being on the tension side of the deformity, there is abundant skin for closure in a tension-free manner (**Fig. 7**).

ARTHROSCOPIC MEDIAL APPROACH TO THE SUBTALAR JOINT

Subtalar arthroscopy is becoming increasingly popular for treatment of a myriad of hindfoot pathologic conditions. Possible indications include investigation of possible articular damage, infection, biopsy, management of sinus tarsi syndrome, loose body removal, arthrodesis, and arthroscopically assisting calcaneal fracture fixation.[12–15] Mekhail and colleagues[16] examined the possibility of the use of a medial portal for access to the subtalar joint in 12 cadavers. They found that a

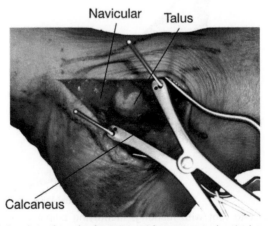

Fig. 4. The medial view into the subtalar joint, with unprepared articular surfaces. The tibialis posterior tendon has been excised, and 2-mm Kirschner wires have been passed into the sustentaculum tali and the talar body and distracted using the Hintermann wire distractor.

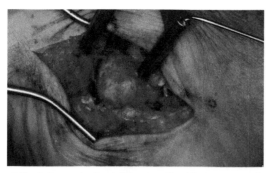

Fig. 5. Distraction of the talar navicular joint using the Hintermann wire distractor.

medial portal gave good visualization of the posterior subtalar joint. The technique of the medial portal consisted of the palpation of the sustentaculum tali and a small stab incision, followed by a sharp trocar to penetration of the deep fascia. This portal was usually at the upper border of the extensor digitorum brevis. At this point, the sharp trocar was replaced by a blunt trocar, which was then introduced in a posterior direction angled 45° to the lateral border of the foot (sagittal plane).[16] Lui[17] reported a case series of 3 patients, where he describes access to the foot and ankle arthroscopists "no-man's land," through a posteromedial portal and a separate medial tarsal tunnel portal. Lui described the placement of a Kirschner wire through a separate lateral portal into the tarsal canal under arthroscopic guidance, pointing toward the medial malleolar tip exiting at the dorsal-distal corner of the medial end of the tarsal canal just behind the sustentaculum tali. At this point, the portal tract is above the flexor hallux longus tendon and the medial plantar nerve. The medial tarsal canal portal was made over this wire. This portal was further studied by a follow-up cadaveric study by Lui and colleagues.[18] Shi and Weinraub[19] compared using medial arthroscopy with open methods for double fusion of the hindfoot. They found a reduced tourniquet time and time to union in the arthroscopic patients compared with the open procedures. Of interest, however, arthroscopy was only performed following the open access to the posterior tibial tendon sheath in all cases.

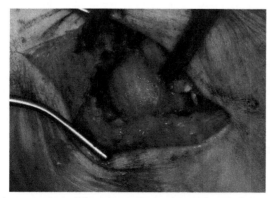

Fig. 6. The ease of preparation of the talar navicular joint through the medial approach and the calcaneocuboid joint visualization in the depth of the surgical wound.

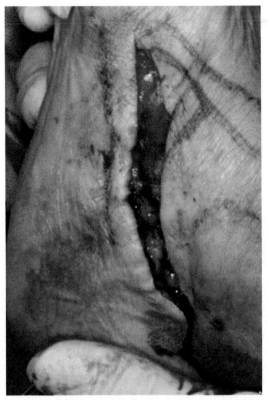

Fig. 7. The wound after deformity correction and before closure. The skin is abundant because of the incision being made on the tension side of the deformity.

VASCULAR RISKS OF MEDIAL APPROACH TO SUBTALAR JOINT

Galli and colleagues[9] reported in a cadaveric study that the neurovascular bundle was a safe distance (21 mm) from the medial approach incision for the subtalar joint. Phisitkul and colleagues,[20] however, relayed concerns in regards to the talar body blood supply with the medial approach. During a cadaveric study, the investigators randomized the specimens to either a single medial incision approach or the traditional 2-incision approach for a triple hindfoot fusion. They found that both approaches could result in substantial disruption of the main blood supply to the talus. The single-medial-incision approach consistently disrupted most of the blood supply to the talar body, whereas the 2-incision approach caused various degrees of vascular disruption to the talar head and neck. Surprisingly, talar osteonecrosis has not been reported in any medial approach clinical studies for hindfoot fusion. This may be the result of a continued blood supply from the calcaneum traversing the fusion site. If this is the case, the medial approach if used for nonfusion surgery may prove a risk for osteonecrosis of the talar body.

RESULTS OF MEDIAL APPROACH HINDFOOT FUSION

In an attempt to attain similar outcomes to the 2-incision triple arthrodesis and achieve an improved complication profile, numerous biomechanical and cadaveric studies have explored the imparted stability on the hindfoot for each fused joint, with the talonavicular joint proving consistently to be the key to hindfoot motion.[21–23] Wülker and colleagues[21] demonstrated a 75% reduction in subtalar joint movement following arthrodesis of the talonavicular joint in cadaveric models. Wülker and colleagues also stated that fusion of the calcaneocuboid joint had no significant influence on the hindfoot motion in the setting of a double (talo-navicular and subtalar) joint fusion. These findings led to several surgeons looking at the efficacy of the double arthrodesis for the treatment of rigid hindfoot deformity.[24]

The single medial incision was assessed by Jeng and colleagues[3] in the context of performing a triple arthrodesis. They looked at the joint surface preparation possible through the medial approach and confirmed that greater than 90% of both subtalar and talonavicular joints could be prepared. This rate was comparable to the standard 2-incision approach often used for a triple arthrodesis. Of interest, they also found that 90% of the calcaneocuboid joint could also be accessed.

With both the subtalar and the talonavicular joints being shown to be safely acces-sible from a single medial incision,[4,9] the procedure lends itself to patients who are deemed high risk for wound complications: patients who suffer from diabetes, rheu-matoid, the elderly, or those with a severe deformity and deficient lateral skin.[25–27] Bril-hault described his outcomes in 14 feet in a patient cohort whereby lateral wound breakdown was deemed probable.[26] With an average follow-up of greater than 20 months, he demonstrated significant radiographic correction and no evidence of wound breakdown. At final follow-up, no patients reported symptoms from their native calcaneocuboid joint. It should be noted that peroneal lengthening was performed as standard via a separate posterolateral incision. Anand and colleagues[28] have also published their results of the medial approach, with a cohort of 18 feet followed up for 2 years. Patient satisfaction was 78%, and all radiographic measures improved significantly. Unfortunately, however, malunion rates and nonunion rates were found to be 12.5% and 11%, respectively. Because of the high complication rate, they did not feel they could recommend the operative technique. Another study, performed in 2006 by Jackson and colleagues,[5] reported improved union rates (100%) with a mean time to union of just more than 5 months. Similar to Brilhault's work, they also reported no issues with wound healing or breakdown. Later work by both Knupp and colleagues[1] and Weinraub and colleagues[29] also report 100% union rates with no wound complications.

More recent studies have undertaken direct comparison of the double arthrodesis via a medial approach compared with a traditional, 2-incision, triple arthrodesis. In 2014, Galli and colleagues[30] performed a retrospective level 3 study comparing the cost and efficacy of the 2 techniques. In a 4-surgeon series, they analyzed hardware cost and procedure time. There was no significant difference with regards to the de-mographics of each group. Time spent in theater was significantly lower in the double-arthrodesis group (106 $\pm$ 31 minutes) compared with the triple procedure (127 $\pm$ 23 minutes). The mean implant cost was also significantly different with the double fusion being on average more than $1700 cheaper. No clinical or radiographic outcomes were assessed. The following year, DeVries and Scharer[31] also published work comparing the 2 techniques. Their data are weakened somewhat by having mixed single- and 2-incision approaches to their double-arthrodesis patients, but con-clusions can still be drawn. Using radiographic outcomes, they wanted to compare the corrective power of each technique. Both fusion types attained significant correction from the preoperative radiographs, and neither fusion type was shown to be more corrective than the other. Of note, they experienced one nonunion of a triple arthrodesis. They state their study adds to the body of evidence advocating a medial approach to a double arthrodesis in the treatment of fixed hindfoot deformity.

Because of the potential risk of iatrogenic injury to the deltoid fibers with the medial approach, Hyer and colleagues[32] proposed a study comparing postoperative ankle valgus for triple- (n = 62) and double-arthrodesis (n = 16) patients. Although there was no difference between the groups' age, sex, body mass index, or laterality, there was a significant difference in mean follow-up with the triple arthrodesis at 17 months and the doubles at 8.75 months. Contrary to their hypothesis, those undergoing triple fusion were 3.6 times more likely to have postoperative valgus ankle alignment compared with those in the medial double-arthrodesis group.

Rausch and colleagues[33] compared 3 approaches for tibiotalocalcaneal arthrodesis, assessing the medial and posterior approaches as compared with the traditional transfibular approach. Arterial structures were least compromised by the transfibular approach. The medial approach had the highest risk of nerve injury, and the venous structures were at their highest risk of all 3 approaches. The proportions of cartilage-debrided joint surfaces of the tibia in the ankle joint, and of the talus and the calcaneus in the subtalar joint, did not differ notably. The proportions of debrided surfaces of the talus in the ankle joint differed notably among the 3 approaches, with the medial approach being inferior to the transfibular approach.

SUMMARY

The medial approach for the subtalar joint provides excellent access to the subtalar joint. The current evidence shows its successful use in subtalar joint fusion combined with talonavicular joint fusion, especially with hindfoot valgus deformity. The medial approach allows adequate correction of deformity and can be easily extended to fuse adjacent joints and to perform additional procedures such as tendon transfer surgery. Complications are reportedly low, with no wound problems or nerve injuries, in contrast to the traditional lateral approach.

REFERENCES

1. Knupp M, Schuh R, Stufkens SA, et al. Subtalar and talonavicular arthrodesis through a single medial approach for the correction of severe planovalgus deformity. J Bone Joint Surg Br 2009;91(5):612–5.
2. Child BJ, Hix J, Catanzariti AR, et al. The effect of hindfoot realignment in triple arthrodesis. J Foot Ankle Surg 2009;48(3):285–93.
3. Jeng CL, Vora AM, Myerson MS. The medial approach to triple arthrodesis. Indications and technique for management of rigid valgus deformities in high-risk patients. Foot Ankle Clin 2005;10(3):515–21, vi–vii.
4. Jeng CL, Tankson CJ, Myerson MS. The single medial approach to triple arthrodesis: a cadaver study. Foot Ankle Int 2006;27(12):1122–5.
5. Jackson WF, Tryfonidis M, Cooke PH, et al. Arthrodesis of the hindfoot for valgus deformity. An entirely medial approach. J Bone Joint Surg Br 2007;89(7):925–7.
6. Saville P, Longman CF, Srinivasan SC, et al. Medial approach for hindfoot arthrodesis with a valgus deformity. Foot Ankle Int 2011;32(8):818–21.
7. Krahenbuhl N, Horn-Lang T, Hintermann B, et al. The subtalar joint: a complex mechanism. EFORT Open Rev 2017;2(7):309–16.
8. Maceira E, Monteagudo M. Subtalar anatomy and mechanics. Foot Ankle Clin 2015;20(2):195–221.
9. Galli MM, Scott RT, Bussewitz B, et al. Structures at risk with medial double hindfoot fusion: a cadaveric study. J Foot Ankle Surg 2014;53(5):598–600.

10. Milner CE, Soames RW. The medial collateral ligaments of the human ankle joint: anatomical variations. Foot Ankle Int 1998;19(5):289–92.
11. Boss AP, Hintermann B. Anatomical study of the medial ankle ligament complex. Foot Ankle Int 2002;23(6):547–53.
12. Tasto JP. Arthroscopy of the subtalar joint and arthroscopic subtalar arthrodesis. Instr Course Lect 2006;55:555–64.
13. Gavlik JM, Rammelt S, Zwipp H. Percutaneous, arthroscopically-assisted osteosynthesis of calcaneus fractures. Arch Orthop Trauma Surg 2002;122(8):424–8.
14. Rammelt S, Gavlik JM, Barthel S, et al. The value of subtalar arthroscopy in the management of intra-articular calcaneus fractures. Foot Ankle Int 2002;23(10): 906–16.
15. Parisien JS, Vangsness T. Arthroscopy of the subtalar joint: an experimental approach. Arthroscopy 1985;1(1):53–7.
16. Mekhail AO, Heck BE, Ebraheim NA, et al. Arthroscopy of the subtalar joint: establishing a medial portal. Foot Ankle Int 1995;16(7):427–32.
17. Lui TH. Medial subtalar arthroscopy. Foot Ankle Int 2012;33(11):1018–23.
18. Lui TH, Chan LK, Chan KB. Medial subtalar arthroscopy: a cadaveric study of the tarsal canal portal. Knee Surg Sports Traumatol Arthrosc 2013;21(6):1279–82.
19. Shi E, Weinraub GM. Arthroscopic medial approach for modified double arthrodesis of the foot. J Foot Ankle Surg 2017;56(1):167–70.
20. Phisitkul P, Haugsdal J, Vaseenon T, et al. Vascular disruption of the talus: comparison of two approaches for triple arthrodesis. Foot Ankle Int 2013;34(4): 568–74.
21. Wülker N, Stukenborg C, Savory KM, et al. Hindfoot motion after isolated and combined arthrodeses: measurements in anatomic specimens. Foot Ankle Int 2000;21(11):921–7.
22. Astion DJ, Deland JT, Otis JC, et al. Motion of the hindfoot after simulated arthrodesis. J Bone Joint Surg Am 1997;79(2):241–6.
23. O'Malley MJ, Deland JT, Lee KT. Selective hindfoot arthrodesis for the treatment of adult acquired flatfoot deformity: an in vitro study. Foot Ankle Int 1995;16(7): 411–7.
24. Sammarco VJ, Magur EG, Sammarco GJ, et al. Arthrodesis of the subtalar and talonavicular joints for correction of symptomatic hindfoot malalignment. Foot Ankle Int 2006;27(9):661–6.
25. Philippot R, Wegrzyn J, Besse JL. Arthrodesis of the subtalar and talonavicular joints through a medial surgical approach: a series of 15 cases. Arch Orthop Trauma Surg 2010;130(5):599–603.
26. Brilhault J. Single medial approach to modified double arthrodesis in rigid flatfoot with lateral deficient skin. Foot Ankle Int 2009;30(1):21–6.
27. Catanzariti AR, Adeleke AT. Double arthrodesis through a medial approach for end-stage adult-acquired flatfoot. Clin Podiatr Med Surg 2014;31(3):435–44.
28. Anand P, Nunley JA, DeOrio JK. Single-incision medial approach for double arthrodesis of hindfoot in posterior tibialis tendon dysfunction. Foot Ankle Int 2013;34(3):338–44.
29. Weinraub GM, Schuberth JM, Lee M, et al. Isolated medial incisional approach to subtalar and talonavicular arthrodesis. J Foot Ankle Surg 2010;49(4):326–30.
30. Galli MM, Scott RT, Bussewitz BW, et al. A retrospective comparison of cost and efficiency of the medial double and dual incision triple arthrodeses. Foot Ankle Spec 2014;7(1):32–6.
31. DeVries JG, Scharer B. Hindfoot deformity corrected with double versus triple arthrodesis: radiographic comparison. J Foot Ankle Surg 2015;54(3):424–7.

32. Hyer CF, Galli MM, Scott RT, et al. Ankle valgus after hindfoot arthrodesis: a radiographic and chart comparison of the medial double and triple arthrodeses. J Foot Ankle Surg 2014;53(1):55–8.
33. Rausch S, Loracher C, Frober R, et al. Anatomical evaluation of different approaches for tibiotalocalcaneal arthrodesis. Foot Ankle Int 2014;35(2):163–7.

Open Technique for In Situ Subtalar Fusion

Stephan H. Wirth, MD*, Stefan M. Zimmermann, MD, Arnd F. Viehöfer, MD, Dipl. Phys

KEYWORDS

• Arthrodesis • Subtalar • Hindfoot

KEY POINTS

- The indication for isolated subtalar fusion concerns subtalar pathologies not manageable by adequate conservative measures.
- The technique has found a widely recognized acceptance and pertains to the orthopedic surgeon armamentarium.
- Isolated subtalar arthritis, either primary or secondary to trauma or inflammatory diseases, is a frequent indication for subtalar fusion.
- Other indications encompass adjacent subtalar joint degeneration after ankle fusion or endoprosthetic ankle joint replacement, painful subtalar instability, and postinfectious arthritis and rheumatoid arthritis.
- Subtalar fusion may be required in patients suffering from talocalcaneal coalition and hindfoot deformities.

INTRODUCTION

Generally speaking, the indication for isolated subtalar fusion concerns subtalar pathologies not manageable by adequate conservative measures. Throughout the past decades, the technique has found a widely recognized acceptance and pertains to the orthopedic surgeon armamentarium.

Isolated subtalar arthritis, either primary or secondary to trauma or inflammatory diseases, is a frequent indication for subtalar fusion. Other indications encompass adjacent subtalar joint degeneration after ankle fusion or endoprosthetic ankle joint replacement, painful subtalar instability, postinfectious arthritis, and rheumatoid arthritis. In addition, subtalar fusion may be required in patients suffering from talocalcaneal coalition and hindfoot deformities, for example, acquired flatfoot deformity secondary to posterior tibial tendon dysfunction.[1–10]

Disclosure: The authors have nothing to confirm.
Department of Orthopedics, Balgrist University Hospital, Forchstrasse 340, Zürich 8008, Switzerland
* Corresponding author.
E-mail address: Stephan.wirth@balgrist.ch

Foot Ankle Clin N Am 23 (2018) 461–474
https://doi.org/10.1016/j.fcl.2018.04.003
1083-7515/18/© 2018 Elsevier Inc. All rights reserved.

The primary aims of isolated subtalar in situ arthrodesis are pain relief and stabilization of the hindfoot. Correction of hindfoot deformity improves hindfoot biomechanics and maintains ankle and midfoot function.[11,12] The first description of subtalar arthrodesis dates back to 1912 and was published by van Stockum.[13] Since then, numerous reports have been published on surgical techniques, fixation methods, functional outcome, fusion rate, and biomechanical considerations. Good overall functional outcome and high fusion rates have been reported for isolated subtalar fusion.

PREOPERATIVE ASSESSMENT
Anatomic and Biomechanical Aspects

Understanding the biomechanics and anatomy of the talocalcaneal subtalar joint is necessary to obtain appropriate positioning of the subtalar joint when performing an arthrodesis.[14–17] The subtalar joint consists of three articulations which are formed by the anterior, middle and posterior facets of the talus and its corresponding facets of the calcaneus, navicular, and calcaneonavicular ligament. They are separated by the sinus tarsi and the tarsal canal.[18] The distinctive joint composition and orientation of the joints enables motion in 3 planes (inversion/eversion, flexion/extension, and abduction/adduction).[14,19,20] Understanding of the biomechanical relationship between hindfoot motion and the triaxial motion of the foot is mandatory in hindfoot surgery.[18] Eversion of the hindfoot allows increased motion in the talonavicular and calcaneocuboid joints as the axis of these joints are aligned in parallel.[21] This allows the foot to adjust to uneven ground during heel strike.[11,14,22] An inversion of the hindfoot during the stance phase locks the transverse joints due to the nonparallel joint axis. This provides a rigid lever arm and permits forward motion. The transversal joints are unlocked when the foot is not loaded. This allows smooth transition from heel strike to the stance phase.[14,20,23,24] If the subtalar joint is fused in too much inversion, however, midfoot flexibility is impaired, which may result in overload of the lateral border of the foot.

Patient History and Clinical Examination

Careful patient history is mandatory. Symptoms of subtalar joint disease include lateral ankle pain, difficulty walking on uneven ground, and pain within or around the sinus tarsi, which is increased by hindfoot inversion and eversion.[1,14] Assessment of the hindfoot axis and the foot arc in the upright standing position of the patient is important. Adult flatfoot deformity with painful posterior tibial tendon insufficiency and overload of the subtalar joint may be aggravated or associated with subfibular impingement and can mimic degeneration of the talocalcaneal joint. Furthermore, pes cavovarus is known to affect the peroneal tendons, which may be clinically mistaken for subtalar joint degeneration[25] (**Fig. 1**). In this-context, accurate clinical examination is crucial for accurate distinction between joint preserving surgical strategies and joint-sacrificing subtalar fusion.[8,26]

Imaging

Standardized radiograph imaging includes weight-bearing anteroposterior (AP) view, lateral view, and dorsoplantar views. This allows assessment of typical signs of degeneration (eg, joint space narrowing, subchondral sclerosis, osteophyte formation, and subchondral cysts). Furthermore, prior placement of hardware can be clearly visualized in cases of posttraumatic osteoarthrosis after fracture fixation as well as adjacent joint degeneration after tibiotalar fusion. Malalignment of the hindfoot (eg, in conjunction with subfibular impingement) may be appreciated in the AP view, and pes cavovarus/pes planovalgus deformity can be detected in the lateral projection. Hindfoot

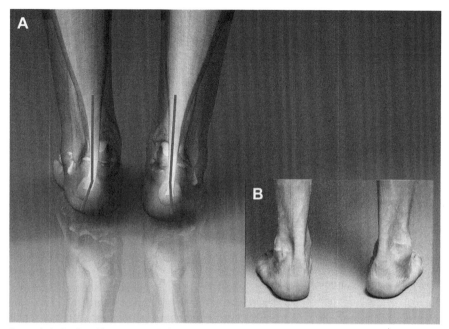

Fig. 1. (A) The hindfoot axis is defined as the angle that is formed by the axis of the calcaneus and the axis of the Achilles tendon. Normal angles range from 0° to 10°. More then 10° is pathologic valgus. Below 0° is varus. Any varus is pathologic. (B) Hindfoot varus.

alignment views or long axial views are recommended for evaluation of the hindfoot axis.[27] The susceptibility of the results to changes in rotation during image generation is described by Buck and colleagues,[27] and further studies have demonstrated that incorrect positioning of the foot during examination may lead to substantial measurement errors.[28] Therefore, care needs to be taken when interpreting the results of an examination in terms of evaluating the position of the foot on plain films. In a phantom study Sutter and colleagues[28] found that 3-D hindfoot alignment measurements based on biplanar radiographs were independent of foot positioning during image acquisition and reader independent. The same group stated the 3-D measurements substantially more precise than the standard radiographic measurements.[28]

MRI

MRI scans of the hindfoot allow assessment of the cartilaginous structures and, therefore, degeneration of the subtalar joint. Due to its accurate depiction of soft-tissue structures (eg, cartilage, tendon, ligaments, and capsules) and specific intraosseous alterations (eg, cysts and bone marrow edema), MRI has gained increased diagnostic importance in daily practice. This is particularly helpful in distinguishing between subtalar degeneration itself and pathologies that mimic subtalar pathologies, as described previously.[25] Moreover, fibrotic (or osseous) coalitions can be readily identified. Finally, MRI scans may be of value in cases of infection to detect osteomyelitis or a remaining sequester.

Computed Tomography

Computed tomography (CT) scans are helpful for assessing bone configuration, the degree of degeneration, and orientation of the hindfoot. Because clinical and conventional radiographic assessment of the subtalar joint is difficult, CT is valuable for evaluation of subtalar joint stability and the exact morphology of hindfoot deformities and is especially helpful to detect bony tarsal coalition.[29] In this context, interesting work regarding orientation of the subtalar joint using full weight-bearing CT scans has recently been published.[29–33]

Diagnostic/Therapeutic Infiltration

Radiographically guided infiltration of the subtalar joint by means of local anesthetics (diagnostic), or mixtures of local anesthetics in combination with steroids (diagnostic and therapeutic with ropivacaine, 2%, and triamcort, 40 mg) is an established method to help to distinguish between subtalar joint pathology and extra-articular sources of pain, for example, tendinopathy of the peroneal tendons.

IN SITU SUBTALAR FUSION—OPERATIVE TECHNIQUE

Once thorough conservative therapy for isolated subtalar pathology has failed, surgical treatment, that is, subtalar arthrodesis, is warranted. The following description of the surgical technique delineates the authors' preferred technique for in situ subtalar fusion.

Patient Positioning and Setup

The patient is positioned supine. The heel is at the distal edge of the operating table for better access to the entry points of implants through the posterior aspect of the heel. If necessary, a cushion is placed under the ipsilateral buttock to better internally rotate the affected leg and provide a better overview of the lateral hindfoot (**Figs. 2** and **3**). The method of anesthesia may vary; however, the procedure is mostly performed under popliteal nerve block in the hospital. In general, blood loss is minimal and a tourniquet is not routinely used. If necessary, a supramalleolar Esmarch bandage is applied in regional anesthesia. If total or spinal anesthesia is performed, a pneumatic tourniquet may be placed on the thigh as close as possible to the groin (see **Fig. 3**). A second-generation cephalosporin is administered as antibiotic prophylaxis 20 minutes before incision. After scrubbing, the leg is draped just below the knee. This enables autologous bone grafting from the proximal tibia if required.

Incision

A lateral subfibular approach is used. Marking of anatomic landmarks is recommended for better orientation. The incision should be marked as well (**Fig. 4**): it starts

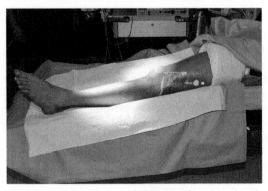

Fig. 2. The patient is positioned supine. A cushion is placed under the ipsilateral hip to slightly invert the leg for better exposure of the lateral hindfoot.

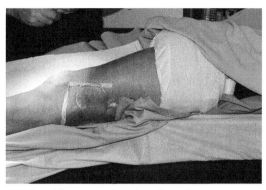

Fig. 3. A tourniquet is placed but not routinely inflamed.

from the distal tip of the fibula parallel to the sole of the foot and extends approximately 3 cm anteriorly to the base of the fourth metatarsal/anterior process of the calcaneus. The skin should be incised carefully by blunt dissection to avoid the underlying branches of the sural nerve.

Approach

The subcutaneous tissue is bluntly dissected in line with the skin incision. Excessive soft tissue dissection should be avoided to prevent postoperative wound breakdown. Great attention is paid to the peroneal tendons. The tendon sheath is left intact. The tendons need to be identified and retracted first by a Langenbeck retractor and later with a Hohmann retractor for proper preparation of the posterior facet. The fat pad in front of the sinus tarsi is mobilized from the fascia of the extensor digitorum brevis muscle in a caudal to cranial fashion and kept in intact (**Fig. 5**). It can be used as a wound cover during closure. The muscle is not routinely dissected in a standardized subtalar fusion.

Next, the tarsal sinus is exposed, and the joint capsule of the subtalar is identified (**Fig. 6**). The joint capsule is horizontally incised and the posterior facet of the calcaneus and the corresponding talar joint surface should become visible. The cervical ligaments are not routinely dissected because blood supply of the calcaneus should be

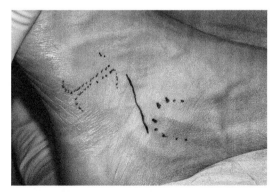

Fig. 4. View of the lateral hindfoot with outlined landmarks. (*Bold dotted line*) Tip of fibula. (*Thin dotted line*) calcaneocuboid joint. (*Solid line*) skin incision.

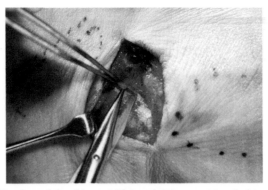

Fig. 5. Blunt mobilization of the sinus tarsi fat pad. It is recommended to save the fat pad to use it for wound closure. Beneath the Langenbeck retractor the peroneal tendons are protected. Left above the forceps is the fascia of extensor digitorum brevis muscle, which is left intact.

tried to be preserved. Dissection of the cervical ligaments, however, may become necessary during the course of the procedure for better visibility. A Hohmann retractor is inserted into the joint capsule in front of the posterior facet aiming medially to retract any soft tissue within the sinus tarsi. A laminar spreader is inserted on the lateral edge as far posteriorly as possible and the subtalar joint is distracted. An excellent view of the subtalar joint should now be obtained.

In cases of severe destruction of the subtalar joint, for example, postinfection, posttrauma, severe osteoarthritis, revision cases, and coalition, it may be difficult to identify the joint. In these cases, the use of intraoperative radiograph/fluoroscopy is helpful to identify the joint and save time.

Joint Preparation

The lateral aspect of the subtalar joint should be débrided. A sharp osteotome, approximately 10 mm in width, is used (**Fig. 7**). The freed cartilage is removed using a small rongeur or sharp curette. The more cartilage is removed, the deeper the laminar spreader can be inserted and the better the subtalar joint can be distracted (**Fig. 8**). The removal of cartilage must be as thorough as possible. This step is essential because it promotes healing of the arthrodesis site. Once cartilage cannot be

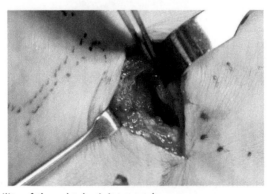

Fig. 6. Good visibility of the subtalar joint capsule.

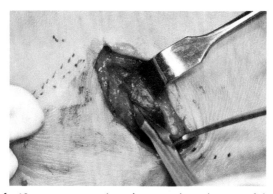

Fig. 7. Insertion of a 10-mm osteotomy into the anterolateral aspect of the subtalar joint. As the cartilage is removed, the distraction of the joint will proceed better. With the osteotome used as a lever arm the joint can be distracted and gains more space to easily insert the laminar spreader.

removed anymore, the laminar spreader is moved to the proximal aspect of the posterior facet. To facilitate this, the osteotome can be left inside the joint to maintain distraction and to allow the insertion of the laminar spreader in the new position. To reach the medial aspect of the joint, a curved osteotome of approximately 5 mm width is useful. Great care is taken not to harm the medial neurovascular structures and tendons (flexor hallucis longus tendon and posterior tibial tendon). To remove the loose cartilage of the medial aspect of the joint, a curved sharp curette is helpful. In addition, regular low-pressure irrigation helps to remove loose cartilage pieces and, especially when not using a tourniquet, helps to identify areas not yet liberated from cartilage. As discussed previously, meticulous cartilage removal is mandatory because improper joint preparation constitutes a relevant risk factor for nonunion. Bone grafting is not routinely performed. If cysts or large bone defects are present, bone grafting is performed. For this purpose, cancellous bone is harvested from either the proximal or distal tibia. Prior to bone grafting, the cysts are débrided and freshened by means of a 2.0-mm drill bit. Next, the denuded facets are cracked open (both talar side and calcaneal side). Proper and regular drill holes within a distance and depth of

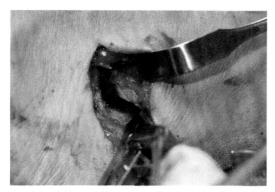

Fig. 8. The laminar spreader is inserted into the subtalar joint. Good visibility of the anterolateral part of the posterior facet. Posterior to the laminar spreader the peroneal tendons are protected.

approximately 2 mm to 3 mm each are placed. Care is taken to perforate the subchondral plate. Alternatively, a small curved osteotome, known from the arthroscopic subtalar fusion technique, may be used to perforate the subchondral plate. The advantage of using the curved osteotome is the absence of heat generation, which may occur when using the drill bit.

Fixation

Fluoroscopy is installed to obtain a true lateral view. The affected leg is elevated and positioned within the fluoroscopy beam. The entry point of the first screw is identified at the posterior aspect of the heel. It is crucial to anticipate the position of the second screw especially in small patients, so that 2 screws aiming preferably perpendicular to the posterior facet can be inserted safely. The foot is held in 5° hindfoot valgus as well as maximal dorsiflexion to compress the fusion site making use of the windlass mechanism by dorsiflexing the great toe (**Fig. 9**). Care is taken that any varus alignment is avoided. A step incision over the calcaneal bone is performed. Skin and subcutaneous tissue are bluntly dissected with a clamp. The first drilling is performed using a 3.2-mm drill bit. The orientation of the drilling is checked under fluoroscopy (**Fig. 10**). The use of an aiming device[34] has demonstrated no advantages in screw positioning in the past but revealed an increased risk of harming the anterior neurovascular structures, which is why it has been abandoned in the authors' clinic. Advantages in reducing radiation time, however, were recorded in the study. The direction is starting posterior inferior at the calcaneus, preferably perpendicular to the posterior facet and to the body of the talus aiming toward the second ray (**Fig. 11**). For use of a fully threaded 6.5-mm cancellous lag screw, a second glide hole is drilled just past the subchondral plate of the posterior facet with a 4.5 mm drill bit. The length of the screw is determined and the screw is inserted under compression of the posterior facet. Under fluoroscopy, an AP view is obtained to control the location of the screw in the frontal plane. A second lag screw is inserted parallel to the first screw. The entry point is at a distance of approximately 1 cm to 2 cm above the first screw but still below the insertion of Achilles tendon. A third (locking) screw is inserted to obtain rotational stability. This screw is aimed from the lateral border of the calcaneus approximately 1 cm posterior to the calcaneocuboid joint toward the talar head in an oblique way. Position and length of the screws are controlled by fluoroscopy in the frontal and sagittal plane. Correct compression of the subtalar joint is verified by fluoroscopy using the lateral view.

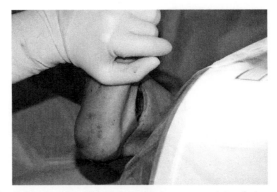

Fig. 9. The foot is elevated and positioned to obtain a proper lateral view using fluoroscopy. The windlass mechanism positions and compresses the subtalar joint. Therefore, the plantar fascia is tensioned by dorsal extension in the metatarsophalangeal (MTP) I and ankle joint.

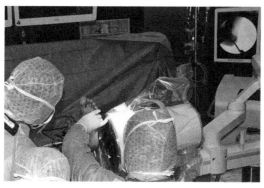

Fig. 10. Under fluoroscopy, the drilling is performed to control direction. To gain compression to the posterior facet the drilling should aim perpendicular to the posterior facet.

Wound Closure

Multiple irrigations of the wounds and meticulous hemostasis are performed. If the peroneal tendon sheath has been opened during the approach, it is sutured using single stitches with Monocryl 3-0 thread (Ethicon, Norderstedt, Germany). The fat pad is reduced over the sinus tarsi und fixed in place with a Monocryl 3-0 thread (Ethicon) (**Fig. 12**). Further irrigation of the wound with saline solution is carried out during the layered wound closure. For subcutaneous suture Monocryl 3-0 (Ethicon) is used paying attention to avoid branches of the sural nerve. Skin suture is performed using single, superficial Donati backstitches with Prolene 4-0 (Ethicon) as a thread. Step incisions at the heel are closed by Donati backstitches using Ethilon 2-0 thread (Ethicon). Sterile wound dressing is applied. The lower leg is well padded. Finally, a soft compression is applied using elastic bandages. The lower leg is immobilized by a cushioned splint with the ankle joint in neutral position, and positioned elevated above the heart level.

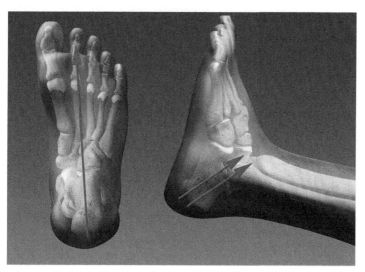

Fig. 11. Red arrows indicate direction of screws. Plantar view (*left*). Aim towards the second toe to be sure not to be too lateral. Lateral view (*right*).

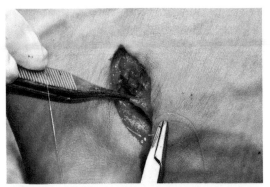

Fig. 12. Refixation of the sinus tarsi fat pad using a resobable 3-0 thread.

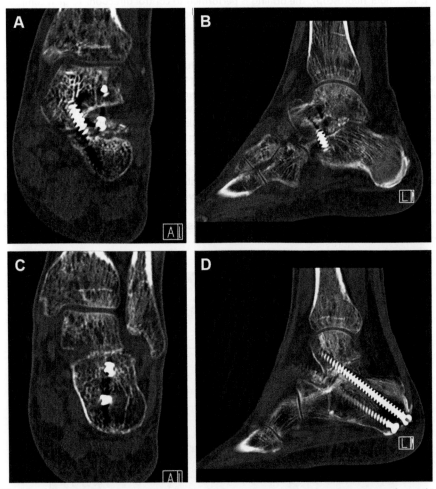

Fig. 13. Postoperative control after 6 weeks. Next to plain radiographs a CT scan is performed to judge osseous fusion. If fusion of more than 50% is reached, weight bearing is increased up to full weight bearing in a knee below walking cast within 4 weeks. (*A*) CT scan coronal plane 6 weeks postoperatively showing medial facet. (*B*) CT scan sagittal plane 6 weeks postoperatively showing medial facet. (*C*) CT scan coronal plane 6 weeks postoperatively showing posterior facet. (*D*) CT scan sagittal plane 6 weeks postoperatively showing posterior facet. A, anterior; L, left.

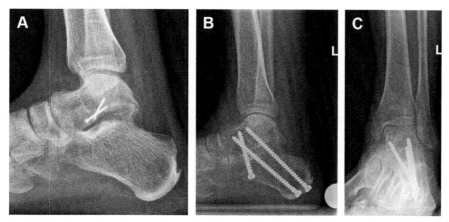

Fig. 14. Twelve-week postoperative control shows fusion, no loosening, and intact implants. (*A*) Preoperative lateral view. (*B*) Twelve-week postoperative lateral view. (*C*) Twelve-week anterior posterior view.

Postoperative Care

Elevation of the leg above heart level should be maintained as long as possible within the first 48 hours postoperatively. Thromboembolic prophylaxis is established for the time of partial weight bearing. Although compression stockings may not have a significant beneficial effect on subjective or objective outcome parameters of patients after hindfoot surgery,[35] compression stockings are nonetheless applied on the contralateral leg to reduce the risk of a thromboembolic event. The first change of wound dressing is carried out 48 hours postoperatively and a below-knee removable cast is applied. The patient is mobilized by physical therapy and instructed to use crutches with partial weight bearing of maximum 15 kg. The patient is discharged when the wounds are dry, pain is controlled by oral analgesics, and secure walking on crutches is commenced. Sutures are removed 2 weeks postoperatively in an outpatient clinic or through a primary care physician; 6 weeks postoperatively, the first postoperative clinical and radiographic follow-up is carried out. Plain radiographs and a CT scan are obtained to judge fusion and screw placement and to exclude screw loosening (**Fig. 13**). Depending on the radiographic evaluation, weight bearing is gradually increased using a walking cast. Full weight bearing should be achieved according to the postoperative regime at 10 weeks after surgery. Final clinical and radiographic follow-up is 12 weeks postoperatively, where plain radiographs are obtained (**Fig. 14**).

SUMMARY

Open subtalar in situ fusion is a well-established surgical procedure, which leads to favorable/excellent fusion rates and functional outcome.[9,15,36–40] Recent studies report favorable to high patient satisfaction.[15,36,40–42] The results seem independent of the fixation method. There are numerous reports of variable numbers of lag screws used in different orientations.[16,39,43–48] Also, staples[10,49] or internal fixation[50] as fixation technique have been reported. Regarding the results of these publications, the fixation techniques for isolated subtalar fusion do not influence outcome and fusion rate. Various different approaches for subtalar fusion are known. A literature review by Tuijthof and colleagues[16] reported possible wound complications and damage of neurovascular structures in all of the evaluated open techniques. Because arthroscopic subtalar fusion is well established in foot and ankle arthroscopy and the results are comparable in terms of fusion rate and functional improvement,[14] an arthroscopically assisted fusion may be considered as an alternative.

REFERENCES

1. Ferrao PN, Saragas NP, Strydom A. Isolated subtalar arthrodesis. JBJS Essent Surg Tech 2016;6:e12–4.
2. Hungerer S, Trapp O, Augat P, et al. Posttraumatic arthrodesis of the subtalar joint - outcome in workers compensation and rates of non-union. Foot Ankle Surg 2011;17:277–83.
3. Ziegler P, Friederichs J, Hungerer S. Fusion of the subtalar joint for post-traumatic arthrosis: a study of functional outcomes and non-unions. Int Orthop 2017;41: 1387–93.
4. Myerson M, Quill GE. Late complications of fractures of the calcaneus. J Bone Joint Surg Am 1993;75A:331–41.
5. Diezi C, Favre P, Vienne P. Primary isolated subtalar arthrodesis: outcome after 2 to 5 years followup. Foot Ankle Int 2008;29:1195–202.
6. Fuhrmann RA, Pillukat T. Subtalar arthrodesis. Oper Orthop Traumatol 2016;28: 177–92 [in German].
7. Myerson MS. Adult acquired flatfoot deformity - treatment of dysfunction of the posterior tibial tendon. J Bone Joint Surg Am 1996;78A:780–92.
8. Kitaoka HB, Patzer GL. Subtalar arthrodesis for posterior tibial tendon dysfunction and pes planus. Clin Orthop Relat Res 1997;(345):187–94.
9. Mann RA, Beaman DN, Horton GA. Isolated subtalar arthrodesis. Foot Ankle Int 1998;19:511–9.
10. Chandler JT, Bonar SK, Anderson R, et al. Results of in situ subtalar arthrodesis for late sequelae of calcaneus fractures. Foot Ankle Int 1999;20:18–24.
11. Astion DJ, Deland JT, Otis JC, et al. Motion of the hindfoot after simulated arthrodesis. J Bone Joint Surg Am 1997;79A:241–6.
12. Jastifer JR, Gustafson PA, Gorman RR. Subtalar arthrodesis alignment: the effect on ankle biomechanics. Foot Ankle Int 2013;34:244–50.
13. van Stockum. Operative behandlung der calcaneus-und talusfraktur. Zentralbl. f. Chir 1912;39:1438–9.
14. Roster B, Kreulen C, Giza E. Subtalar joint arthrodesis: open and arthroscopic indications and surgical techniques. Foot Ankle Clin 2015;20:319–34.
15. Yildirim T, Sofu H, Çamurcu Y, et al. Isolated subtalar arthrodesis. Acta Orthop Belg 2015;81:155–60.
16. Tuijthof GJM, Beimers L, Kerkhoffs GMMJ, et al. Overview of subtalar arthrodesis techniques: options, pitfalls and solutions. Foot Ankle Surg 2010;16:107–16.
17. Inman VT. The joints of the ankle. Baltimore: Williams & Wilkins; 1976.
18. Snedeker JG, Wirth SH, Espinosa N. Biomechanics of the normal and arthritic ankle joint. Foot Ankle Clin 2012;17:517–28.
19. Keefe DT, Haddad SL. Subtalar instability. Etiology, diagnosis, and management. Foot Ankle Clin 2002;7:577–609.
20. Barg A, Tochigi Y, Amendola A, et al. Subtalar instability: diagnosis and treatment. Foot Ankle Int 2012;33:151–60.
21. Elftman H. The transverse tarsal joint and its control. Clin Orthop 1960;16:41–6.
22. Krähenbühl N, Horn-Lang T, Hintermann B, et al. The subtalar joint: a complex mechanism. EFORT Open Rev 2017;2:309–16.
23. Perry J. Anatomy and biomechanics of the hindfoot. Clin Orthop Relat Res 1983;(177):9–15.

24. Mann RA, Haskell A. Biomechanics of the foot and ankle. In: Coughlin M, Mann RA, Saltzmann CL, editors. Manns surgery of the foot and ankle. 8th edition. Philadelphia: Elsevier Health; 2007. p. 3–45.
25. Perera A, Guha A. Clinical and radiographic evaluation of the cavus foot surgical implications. Foot Ankle Clin 2013;18:619–28.
26. Hintermann B. Lateral column lengthening osteotomy of calcaneus. Oper Orthop Traumatol 2015;27:298–307 [in German].
27. Buck FM, Hoffmann A, Mamisch-Saupe N, et al. Hindfoot alignment measurements: rotation-stability of measurement techniques on hindfoot alignment view and long axial view radiographs. AJR Am J Roentgenol 2011;197: 578–82.
28. Sutter R, Pfirrmann CWA, Espinosa N, et al. Three-dimensional hindfoot alignment measurements based on biplanar radiographs: comparison with standard radiographic measurements. Skeletal Radiol 2013;42:493–8.
29. Krähenbühl N, Tschuck M, Bolliger L, et al. Orientation of the subtalar joint. Foot Ankle Int 2015;37:109–14.
30. Apostle KL, Coleman NW, Sangeorzan BJ. Subtalar joint axis in patients with symptomatic peritalar subluxation compared to normal controls. Foot Ankle Int 2014;35:1153–8.
31. Colin F, Lang TH, Zwicky L, et al. Subtalar joint configuration on weightbearing CT scan. Foot Ankle Int 2014;35:1057–62.
32. Probasco W, Haleem AM, Yu J, et al. Assessment of coronal plane subtalar joint alignment in peritalar subluxation via weight-bearing multiplanar imaging. Foot Ankle Int 2015;36:302–9.
33. Hirschmann A, Pfirrmann CWA, Klammer G, et al. Upright cone CT of the hindfoot: comparison of the non-weight-bearing with the upright weight-bearing position. Eur Radiol 2014;24:553–8.
34. Betz M, Wieser K, Vich M, et al. Precision of targeting device for subtalar screw placement. Foot Ankle Int 2012;33:519–23.
35. Grubhofer F, Catanzaro S, Schüpbach R, et al. Compressive stockings after hindfoot and ankle surgery. Foot Ankle Int 2018;39(2):210–8.
36. Easley ME, Trnka H-J, Schon LC, et al. Isolated subtalar arthrodesis. J Bone Joint Surg Am 2000;82:613–24.
37. Flemister AS, Infante AF, Sanders RW, et al. Subtalar arthrodesis for complications of intra-articular calcaneal fractures. Foot Ankle Int 2000;21:392–9.
38. Davies MB, Rosenfeld PF, Stavrou P, et al. A comprehensive review of subtalar arthrodesis. Foot Ankle Int 2007;28:295–7.
39. Haskell A, Pfeiff C, Mann R. Subtalar joint arthrodesis using a single lag screw. Foot Ankle Int 2004;25:774–7.
40. Catanzariti AR, Mendicino RW, Saltrick KR, et al. Subtalar joint arthrodesis. J Am Podiatr Med Assoc 2005;95:34–41.
41. Burton DC, Olney BW, Horton GA. Late results of subtalar distraction fusion. Foot Ankle Int 1998;19:197–202.
42. Huefner T, Thermann H, Geerling J, et al. Primary subtalar arthrodesis of calcaneal fractures. Foot Ankle Int 2001;22:9–14.
43. Hungerer S, Eberle S, Lochner S, et al. Biomechanical evaluation of subtalar fusion: the influence of screw configuration and placement. J Foot Ankle Surg 2013;52:177–83.
44. Matsumoto T, Glisson RR, Reidl M, et al. Compressive force with 2-screw and 3-screw subtalar joint arthrodesis with headless compression screws. Foot Ankle Int 2016;37:1357–63.

45. Boffeli TJ, Reinking RR. A 2-screw fixation technique for subtalar joint fusion: a retrospective case series using a 2-screw fixation construct with operative pearls. J Foot Ankle Surg 2012;51:734–8.

46. Scanlan RL, Burns PR, Crim BE. Technique tip: subtalar joint fusion using a parallel guide and double screw fixation. J Foot Ankle Surg 2010;49:305–9.

47. DeCarbo WT, Berlet GC, Hyer CF, et al. Single-screw fixation for subtalar joint fusion does not increase nonunion rate. Foot Ankle Spec 2010;3:164–6.

48. Gosch C, Verrette R, Lindsey DP, et al. Comparison of initial compression force across the subtalar joint by two different screw fixation techniques. J Foot Ankle Surg 2006;45:168–73.

49. Herrera-Pérez M, Andarcia-Bañuelos C, Barg A, et al. Comparison of cannulated screws versus compression staples for subtalar arthrodesis fixation. Foot Ankle Int 2015;36:203–10.

50. Dennyson WG, Fulford GE. Subtalar arthrodesis by cancellous grafts and metallic internal fixation. J Bone Joint Surg Br 1977;58:507–10.

Subtalar Arthroscopic Fusion

Emilio Wagner, MD[a],*, Rodrigo Melo, MD[b]

KEYWORDS

- Subtalar fusion • Posterior approach • 3 portal technique • Arthroscopic fusion

KEY POINTS

- The subtalar joint is a complex joint involved in human locomotion, essential in shock absorption and propulsion in gait.
- Failure of conservative treatment warrants surgical intervention, where subtalar fusion delivers excellent results when properly aligned.
- Arthroscopic subtalar fusion can deliver faster return to activities and sports, achieving high fusion rates.
- Proper preparation of joint surfaces, excellent hindfoot alignment, and a solid construct are key elements to achieve a successful outcome.

INTRODUCTION

The subtalar joint refers to the joint between the talus and the calcaneus. It is a complex joint, which is involved in human locomotion, playing an important role in shock absorption and propulsion. Subtalar arthrodesis is an accepted surgical treatment of subtalar pathologic condition whereby conservative treatments have failed to provide a successful outcome. Common indications for subtalar fusion are posttraumatic or degenerative arthrosis, arthritis, talocalcaneal coalitions, and complex deformities.[1]

BIOMECHANICS

This joint is designed to provide either a flexible shock absorption construct to the foot or a rigid propulsive one.[2] Every time the subtalar joint is everted, or in valgus, the foot will become a flexible structure because the transverse tarsal joints are unlocked. When the subtalar joint inverts, the transverse tarsal joints lock themselves, and this provides a rigid lever arm, which is beneficial for locomotion.[3] The subtalar joint is

---

Disclosure Statement: The authors have nothing to disclose.
[a] Foot and Ankle Unit, Clinica Alemana, Universidad del Desarrollo, 5951, Vitacura, Vitacura, Santiago 7650568, Chile; [b] Foot and Ankle Unit, Hospital Militar, Universidad de Los Andes, Av. Alcalde Fernando Castillo Velasco 9100, La Reina, Santiago, Chile
* Corresponding author.
E-mail address: ewagner@alemana.cl

foot.theclinics.com

divided by the sinus tarsi, into the talocalcaneonavicular joint anteriorly and talocalcaneal joint posteriorly. This fact explains why just the posterior subtalar facet is visible from the more classic surgical approaches, which do not violate the sinus tarsi.

During locomotion, pronation and supination alternate successively in a harmonious pattern. They are complex triplane movements of the foot, whereby the largest amount of motion occurs at the talonavicular joint followed by the talocalcaneal joint. Fusion of the talonavicular joint completely blocks the motions at the subtalar joint, but in contrast, fusion of the subtalar joint does allow motion at adjacent joints.[2] After simulated arthrodesis of the subtalar joint, the remaining motion has been calculated to be 74% for the talonavicular joint and 44% for the calcaneocuboid joint.[4]

Analyzing subtalar motion, the sagittal plane is the least dominant one, and therefore, subtalar joint pathologic condition may not affect progression of gait. This last mechanical fact explains why the subtalar joint is considered a nonessential joint for gait and posture.[2] Subtalar fusion for pathologic condition unresponsive to conservative treatment will therefore still be one of the treatments of choice, as long it is adequately aligned.

EVALUATION

A detailed history and physical examination must be performed when a patient presents with subtalar pain. Difficulty when walking on uneven grounds is a classic symptom, which is taught but not always present. Pain is typically found in the posterolateral aspect of the hindfoot, close and around the sinus tarsi area, or it can radiate from the posterolateral to the posteromedial aspect, including the posterior aspect of the hindfoot. Rarely, pain will be found at the anterior aspect of the hindfoot, where the ankle joint is assumed to be the source of pain. Motion at the subtalar joint is not easy to examine, because subtalar joint range of motion can be mistaken for ankle joint motion, but contralateral examination can help. Hindfoot alignment is a prerequisite, with the patient standing, from the front and from the posterior aspect. Normal mechanics must be checked; for example, when asking the patient to stand on the tip of the toes, the hindfoot must invert, and when the foot lands on the ground, a smooth eversion and pronation must occur.

Imaging generally includes radiographic imaging of the ankle, besides hindfoot alignment views. In this matter, the authors prefer complete leg standing radiographs, which include the foot. They have been more useful than the classic axial or Saltzman views. Computed tomographic (CT) scan is also useful because it evaluates the extent of the deformity, besides ruling out a coalition. Single-photon emission CT has been in use in the last few years because it allows identifying the source of pain when internal fixation is present, especially in posttraumatic cases whereby the origin of pain is not well defined by conventional imaging methods.

Nonoperative treatment should aim to reduce pain, limiting somehow hindfoot motion. Classic conservative treatments include weight modifications, analgesic medications, subtalar joint injections, shock absorption elements such as shoes or insoles, and special insoles made to limit hindfoot motion.[3] Medially posted insoles can reduce eversion movements with respect to the hindfoot, and therefore, may help in controlling subtalar pain.[5] When conservative treatment fails, a surgical intervention is justified.

INDICATIONS

Subtalar joint fusion is indicated for various conditions that affect the subtalar joint, mainly primary osteoarthritis, inflammatory arthropathy, talocalcaneal coalitions, posttraumatic arthrosis, and acquired flatfoot deformity, the most common ones. A successful subtalar arthrodesis can be obtained through open or arthroscopic approaches. The reason behind trying an arthroscopic approach is to preserve the blood supply to the talus, to reduce postoperative morbidity, and it is hoped, to obtain better results. It was first described in 1985, and later, successful results have been published by others.[6] The time to union and time to return to activities of daily living, sports, and work are shorter after arthroscopic approaches when compared with open ones.[7] Open techniques present risk of wound infection, neurovascular damage, and delayed wound healing, risks which are notoriously diminished by the arthroscopic approach.[1] Having said this, after analyzing union rates and overall complications, there is no proven advantage of one approach over the other.[7] Currently, open approaches would be preferred for conditions with large deformities, significant bone loss of the talus or calcaneus, revision cases with prior surgeries, and nonunions.[3] In most of the cases, with adequate surgical experience, an arthroscopic approach is preferred.

SURGICAL TECHNIQUE

The subtalar joint can be accessed arthroscopically either from the lateral aspect or from the posterior aspect of the joint. For the lateral approach, a 2.7-mm 30° short arthroscope is recommended, using also a small joint shaver as a basic working instrument. The recommended portals for this approach include an anterolateral one placed 1 cm distal and 2 cm anterior to the fibular tip, a middle portal 1 cm anterior to the tip of the fibula over the sinus tarsi, and a posterolateral one 0.5 cm proximal to the fibular tip just lateral to the Achilles tendon[8] (**Figs. 1** and **2**). For the posterior approach, 2 portals can be used, that is, the posterolateral and the posteromedial portals, which are placed at similar points relative to the Achilles tendon at or just proximal to the tip of the fibula. The main difference between the posterior and lateral approach is that this last one is a true arthroscopic approach, in comparison to the posterior approach that starts as an extra-articular approach.

Currently, the authors prefer a posterior arthroscopic approach using 3 portals, using the previously mentioned posterolateral and posteromedial portals plus an accessory sinus tarsi portal, which is useful to introduce a blunt trocar to create space in the joint and to remove the anterior cartilage of the subtalar joint.[9]

The patients are placed in the prone position, with or without a thigh tourniquet. The ankle joint is left at the end of the table to have ample room to perform dorsiflexion by

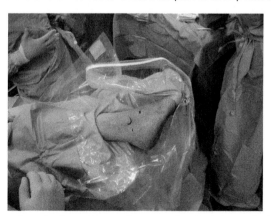

Fig. 1. General setup for subtalar arthroscopic approach, which forms the lateral aspect. The anterolateral and posterolateral portals can be seen marked on the skin.

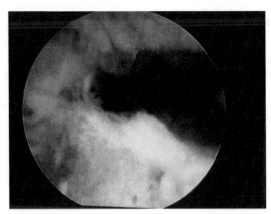

Fig. 2. Intraoperative arthroscopic view from the lateral approach. The lateral aspect of the posterior subtalar facet can be seen.

the surgeon. The operated leg remains elevated in relation to the nonoperated one, to aid fluoroscopic lateral evaluation for subtalar fixation. A support under the ipsilateral iliac crest places the foot in the vertical position. The portals are placed as described elsewhere, at the level of the fibular tip, just lateral and medial to the Achilles tendon. While performing the posterolateral portal, the trocar is pointed to the first interdigital web space. The posterior medial portal is performed following the path of the posterolateral portal to avoid any damage to the medial structures (**Fig. 3**).

The subtalar joint is easily identified by this approach. In patients with severe subtalar osteoarthritis, however, the joint line may be blurred because of a posterior fibrosis, large osteophytes, and severe joint space narrowing. The most important anatomic landmark is the flexor hallucis longus (FHL) tendon, which marks the medial boundary of the working area (**Fig. 4**). Going beyond this structure, that is, medially, is dangerous because of potential risk of injury of the neurovascular structures. The tendon of the FHL is easier to visualize after first identifying the belly of the muscle immediately proximal to the posterior talar process.[10]

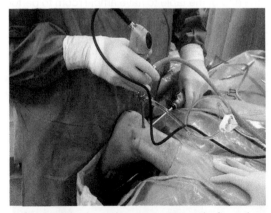

Fig. 3. General setup for the subtalar arthroscopic approach, from the posterior approach. The ankle is hanging from the table margin, so that free joint motion can be obtained. The posterolateral and posteromedial portals are being used.

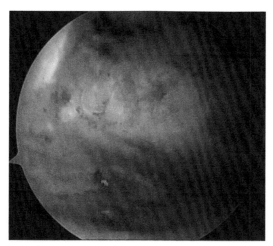

Fig. 4. Intraoperative arthroscopic view from the posterior approach. The posterior aspect of the posterior subtalar facet can be seen. On the upper left margin of the picture, the flexor hallucis longus can be observed.

Visualizing the entire joint space is difficult. Quite often distraction is required to achieve this goal, and the placement of an accessory portal can be useful. For this portal, at the level of the sinus tarsi, a needle is used to locate correctly the entry point. The position of the needle is controlled intra-articularly and from the posterior. Then, a small clamp is used to prepare the entrance of a blunt trocar of a large diameter, for example, 4.0 mm, and to facilitate the distraction and joint preparation. Several distraction methods are available: manual traction, assistant hold, intra-articular trocar, or an external distractor.[10] However, with continuous preparation of the joint surfaces, the joint starts to open up, and no manual or other traction devices are necessary.

Proper removal of cartilage is mandatory. For this purpose, shaver, curettes, and burrs are used.[1] Osteotomes can be used to crack open the subchondral bone areas and to enlarge the surfaces to promote fusion (**Figs. 5** and **6**). When correcting

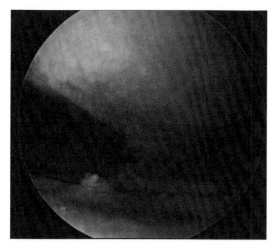

Fig. 5. Intraoperative arthroscopic view from the posterior approach. A chisel is being inserted to perform grooves on the joint surfaces, to improve bone bleeding.

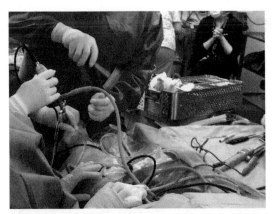

Fig. 6. General setup for subtalar arthroscopic approach. With the help of the assistant, bone grooves are performed using an arthroscopic chisel.

hindfoot deformities, the posterior approach is especially useful, because the prone position helps in achieving a correct alignment of the hindfoot. It is easy to achieve a slight valgus position of the subtalar joint. It has been shown that the ideal position of the subtalar joint is in 5° to 10° of valgus to maximize muscle generating force capacity and muscle lever arm.[11]

When perfect bone adaptation and compression are achieved, no additional grafting material is needed. However, sometimes deformities, larger cavities of the talus, or calcaneus may require additional bone grafting to add stability and a higher probability of bone healing (**Fig. 7**). In a clinical study dealing with hindfoot and ankle arthrodesis, 200 subtalar fusions were studied. The authors found that filling the fusion zone with more than 50% of graft material was associated with significantly higher fusion rates at 24 weeks.[12]

When considering fixation, generally 2 screws are recommended to avoid rotational instability[1] (**Fig. 8**). It is the authors' preference to use 2 screws in a divergent position

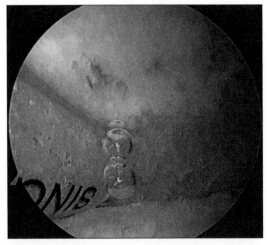

Fig. 7. Intraoperative arthroscopic view from the posterior approach. Bone substitute is being injected into the joint space to fill properly the space.

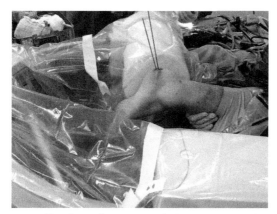

Fig. 8. General setup to allow bone fixation. Axial alignment is checked visually, trying to achieve 5° of hindfoot valgus. A proper lateral hindfoot view is taken to ensure correct position of guide wires, choosing to fix the screw crossing the posterior subtalar joint first. In the picture, just one K wire was left when inserting the posterior screw.

to achieve a stiffer biomechanical construct, which has been proven in the literature[13] (**Fig. 9**). Nevertheless, when performing fixation, the authors strongly recommend placing one screw or its guide wire first if using a cannulated system, and fixing and tightening one screw before inserting the second K wire. The first screw acts as a true compressive screw, and the second screw becomes a stabilizer. Placing 2 K wires at the same time will block any compression provided by the screws and may delay bone healing.

RESULTS

Satisfactory outcomes can be expected in 85% when there is no misalignment present. In cases with misalignment, the rate of success reduces to 65%.[1] Outcomes of fusion rates vary considerable, because many articles used only simple conventional radiographic to assess bony union. Apparently, to consider a fusion to be

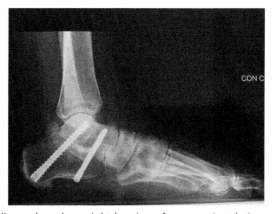

Fig. 9. Lateral radiograph under weight-bearing of same patient being operated. Observe the divergent position of the screws, achieving axial compression with the posterior screw and avoiding rotation with the anterior one.

successful (besides a good clinical result), an osseous bridging between 25% and 49% of the joint surface would suffice.[14] The presence of posttraumatic arthrosis imposes a higher risk of nonunion, for example, as high as 24% in previous calcaneal fractures, probably mediated by local vascular changes and bone defects.[15] Time to union can be as low as 11 weeks, with significant improvements in clinical scores and hindfoot alignment parameters.[7] Most recent published articles show union rates of 95% after an average postoperative time interval of 12 weeks. CT scans are highly reliable in assessing bony union.

COMPLICATIONS

Arthroscopic approaches present more hardware-related complications than open approaches, as it has been shown in the literature.[6,7,16] Sural nerve symptoms can be found in up to 6%, because of the proximity of the posterolateral portal to the sural nerve, which is located 4 mm posterior to the nerve. At risk also are the tibial neurovascular structures, where the posterior bundle is on average 1 cm anterior to the posteromedial portal. The distance between the portal and the tibial nerve has been reported to be 6.4 mm, which illustrates the care that must be taken when positioning this posteromedial portal.[8]

SUMMARY

The posterior arthroscopic approach is a useful method to achieve successful subtalar fusions, with minimal morbidity and high fusion rates. Contraindications for this approach must be considered, because severe misalignments and bone loss present serious difficulties, and an open approach should be considered in these cases. Possible complications to be considered are mainly due to inadequate surgical technique and to proximity to neurovascular structures when placing the arthroscopic portals. It is important to achieve an adequate bone contact at the joint surface to obtain a satisfactory fusion. In appropriate patients, an arthroscopic approach can obtain fast union rates with minimal morbidity and is the preferred technique of the authors.

REFERENCES

1. Tuijthof G, Beimers L, Kerkhoffs G, et al. Overview of subtalar arthrodesis techniques: options, pitfalls and solutions. Foot Ankle Surg 2010;16:107–16.
2. Maceira E, Monteagudo M. Subtalar anatomy and mechanics. Foot Ankle Clin N Am 2015;20:195–221.
3. Roster B, Kreulen C, Giza E. Subtalar joint arthrodesis, open and arthroscopic indications and surgical techniques. Foot Ankle Clin N Am 2015;20:319–34.
4. Astion D, Deland J, Otis J, et al. Motion of the hindfoot after simulated arthrodesis. J Bone Joint Surg Am 1997;79(2):241–6.
5. Kosonen J, Kulmala J, Muller E, et al. Effects of medially posted insoles on foot and lower limb mechanics across walking and running in overpronating men. J Biomech 2017;54:58–63.
6. Vila-Rico J, Mellado-Romero M, Bravo-Gimenez B, et al. Subtalar arthroscopic arthrodesis: technique and outcomes. Foot Ankle Surg 2017;23:9–15.
7. Rungprai C, Phisitkul P, Femino J, et al. Outcomes and complications after open versus posterior arthroscopic subtalar arthrodesis in 121 patients. J Bone Joint Surg Am 2016;98:636–46.
8. Beimers L, Frey C, van Dijk C. Arthroscopy of the posterior subtalar joint. Foot Ankle Clin N Am 2006;11:369–90.

9. Beimers L, Leeuw P, Van Dijk C. A 3-portal approach for arthroscopic subtalar arthrodesis. Knee Surg Sports Traumatol Arthrosc 2009;17:830–4.
10. Lopes R, Andrieu M, Bauer T. Arthroscopic subtalar arthrodesis. Orthop Traumatol Surg Res 2016;102(8S):S311–6.
11. Jastifer J, Gustafson P, Gorman R. Subtalar arthrodesis alignment: the effect on ankle biomechanics. Foot Ankle Int 2013;34(2):244–50.
12. DiGiovanni C, Lin S, Daniels T, et al. The importance of sufficient graft material in achieving foot or ankle fusion. J Bone Joint Surg Am 2016;98:1260–7.
13. Jastifer J, Alrafeek S, Howard P, et al. Biomechanical evaluation of strength and stiffness of subtalar joint arthrodesis screw constructs. Foot Ankle Int 2016;37(4): 419–26.
14. Glazebrook M, Beasley W, Daniels T, et al. Establishing the relationship between clinical outcome and extent of osseous bridging between computed tomography assessment in isolated hindfoot and ankle fusions. Foot Ankle Int 2013;34(12): 1612–8.
15. Ziegler P, Friederichs J, Hungerer S. Fusion of the subtalar joint for post-traumatic arthrosis: a study of functional outcomes and non-unions. Int Orthop 2017;41: 1387–93.
16. Oliva X, Falcao P, Fernandez Cerqueira R, et al. Posterior arthroscopic subtalar arthrodesis: clinical and radiologic review of 19 cases. J Foot Ankle Surg 2017; 56:543–6.

Subtalar Distraction Arthrodesis

Norman Espinosa, MD*, Elena Vacas, MD

KEYWORDS

- Subtalar joint • Subtalar distraction arthrodesis • Achilles tendon lengthening
- Structural bone graft

KEY POINTS

- The subtalar joint can be altered in its anatomy and biomechanical behavior.
- It is important to know how to assess the talar declination angle in order to assess the deformity at the subtalar joint.
- Consider a straight posterior approach to the subtalar joint and remain liberal in the use of z-shaped Achilles tendon lengthening.
- A structural bone graft should be used to elevate the talus.
- Positioning screws should be used to lock the construct.

INTRODUCTION

The subtalar joint is fascinating and is essential in adapting the foot and ankle to different shapes of the ground. However, there are various causes that may irreversibly alter the anatomy and biomechanics of the subtalar joint leading to chronic impairment dysfunction.[1–3] The most important encompass calcaneal fractures, Charcot neuroarthropathy, avascular necrosis of the talus, and status after surgical treatment.[4–6] Iatrogenic causes include nonunion and malunion after subtalar joint arthrodesis. In addition, even congenital causes, for example, residual clubfoot deformities, can end up in a grotesque hindfoot anatomy that affects the subtalar joint.[7,8] In the presence of degenerative diseases, that is, arthrosis, and the indication to embark on surgery, these anatomic alterations become very important and should be taken into consideration.

The loss of height and possibly present lateral, subfibular impingement of the peroneal tendons may occur in the case of malunited calcaneal fractures, iatrogenic and/or congenitally distorted hindfeet as well, resulting in relevant impairment of the patients.

A surgeon needs to anticipate the problems of the subtalar joint and how to correct them properly. An in situ arthrodesis of a malunited calcaneus with massive talar

Disclosure: The authors have nothing to disclose.
Institute for Foot and Ankle Reconstruction, Kappelistrasse 7, Zurich 8002, Switzerland
* Corresponding author.
E-mail address: espinosa@fussinstitut.ch

declination after fracture will never address the accompanying loss of height and sub-fibular impingement.[9]

Therefore, subtalar distraction arthrodesis has become an important technique to address the problem of hindfoot deformity and arthrosis as well. The technique is used to restore height, correct heel width, and eliminate subtalar arthrosis.

INDICATIONS

As pointed out by Myerson,[10] "the indications for a subtalar distraction arthrodesis are fairly specific." They include certain conditions, whereby arthrodesis of the subtalar joint is required but also loss of hindfoot height is present. In those hindfeet, the talar declination might be negative with a consecutive anterior narrowing of the ankle joint. The narrow anterior ankle space could lead to limited dorsiflexion and ankle impingement syndrome (**Fig. 1**). Therefore, ankle range of motion and anterior ankle pain must be assessed. Although Myerson and Quill[11] reported the indications to be (1) loss of heel height >8 mm, (2) anterior ankle impingement due to abnormal talar declination angle, these values were strongly debated by Chandler and colleagues.[4] In patients who do not demonstrate any loss of range of motion or who do not have pain may be candidates for an in situ subtalar arthrodesis. Similar indications were given by Chandler and colleagues,[4] who recommended distraction arthrodesis only in patients with given findings of anterior ankle impingement. However, the biomechanics of the hindfoot will never be restored.

CONTRAINDICATIONS

Patients with impaired vascularity and concomitant brittle or scarred tissue are in danger to develop serious and precarious wound-healing problems.

In the case of talar necrosis, the surgery should be thought through because insertion of a bone graft needs adequate perfusion to allow proper incorporation. If possible, a vascularized medial femoral bone graft can be taken into consideration and connected to the posterior tibial artery.[12] However, the latter requires the presence of an experienced plastic surgeon.

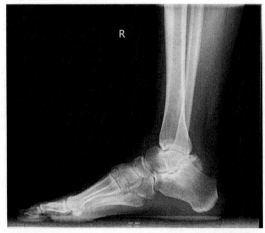

Fig. 1. The narrow anterior part of the ankle joint ends after posterior declination of the talus.

PREPARATION OF SURGERY

Adequate tools and meticulous preparation are absolutely mandatory before starting such a demanding surgery. Otherwise, complications may be encountered during the procedure, which may negatively affect the final clinical outcome.

Standardized radiographs are required. Those radiographs include full weight-bearing dorsoplantar, lateral, anteroposterior, axial, or hindfoot alignment views.

The lateral view allows the evaluation of the talocalcaneal angle, the talar declination angle, and the calcaneal height (**Fig. 2**).

The talocalcaneal angle is formed by the intersection of the central talar axis line with the longitudinal axis line of the calcaneus. Its normal angle value ranges between 25° and 45° (see **Fig. 2**).

The talar declination angle is represented by the intersection of the perpendicular line to the floor and a line perpendicular to the line through the long axis of the talus (see **Fig. 2**).

The calcaneal height is measured from the talar dome to the base of the calcaneus (see **Fig. 2**).

It is recommended to get weight-bearing radiographs of the healthy contralateral side, in order to compare and assess the angles properly.

SURGICAL TECHNIQUE IN DETAIL

The patient is placed in either the lateral decubitus or the prone position (**Fig. 3**). The approach used by the authors is typically vertical. This approach allows closure of the skin, whereas a lateral approach could potentially endanger it.

Usually, the vertical limb of the previous extensile approach is extended proximally. Even if there is any hardware to remove, the authors prefer to retrieve only those implants that are necessary in order to allow firm fixation of the subtalar distraction arthrodesis (**Fig. 4**).

The Authors' Approach

The proximal and vertical skin incision is frequently performed paralateral to the Achilles tendon (**Fig. 5**). The sural nerve is at risk and should be avoided and protected. If

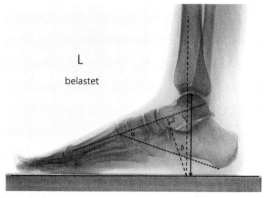

Fig. 2. The lateral weight-bearing view of a left foot. Alpha represents the talocalcaneal angle, which is formed by the intersecting lines of the midline of the talus and the longitudinal axis of the calcaneus. The talar declination angle is formed by the intersection of a perpendicular line to the talar midaxis line and a perpendicular line to the floor (beta angle).

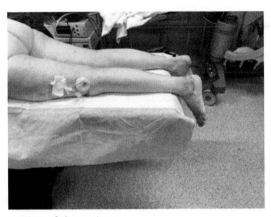

Fig. 3. The prone position of the patient.

there is no chance to preserve it, some surgeons suggest transecting it and burying it more proximally into the muscle belly of the flexor hallucis longus muscle belly.

In the presence of massive talar declination and triceps surae contracture, it might be preferable to add a z-shaped lengthening of the Achilles tendon (**Fig. 6**), which allows a better opening of the subtalar joint and easier handling to insert the bone graft.

Primary Dissection

The first landmark is the posterior calcaneal tuberosity (**Fig. 7**). The lateral wall and small parts of the posteromedial calcaneal wall can be exposed subperiosteally. When there is massive widening of the lateral calcaneal wall present, it is possible to perform an exostectomy through this approach. The exostectomy can be performed using either an osteotome or a saw blade. The authors prefer to use an osteotome. The ostectomy is started on the posterior margin of the tuberosity of the calcaneus inferior to the posterior facet. The whole bone should then be removed. The bone block may be used as autograft for later fixation.

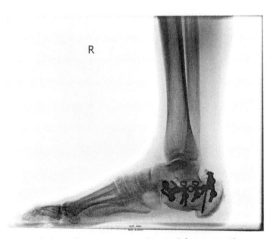

Fig. 4. Posttraumatic condition after a severe calcaneal fracture. Please note the amount of hardware and the potential complications associated with them.

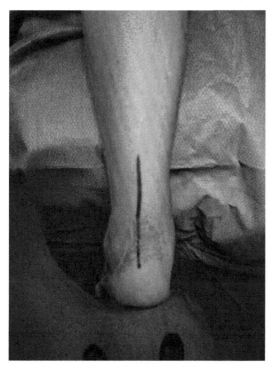

Fig. 5. The incision is made posterolaterally to the Achilles tendon and vertical to ensure proper closure at the end of the surgery.

Intermediate Dissection

The next level is the fat triangle of Kager, which needs to be divided centrally. The authors do not recommend removing of the entire fat pad, because this would impair proper coverage and sealing of the postoperative subtalar wound zone.

Deep Dissection

After dissection of the fat pad, the posterior aspect of the subtalar joint is reached. The posterior surface of the calcaneus helps the surgeon to guide the way until proceeding anteriorly to the posterior part of the subtalar joint. Fluoroscopy assists to identify the posterior facet of the subtalar joint. Direct visualization can be difficult, especially in the presence of massive talar declination. A 10-mm to 15-mm osteotome is introduced, and the level of its subtalar penetration is checked fluoroscopically (**Fig. 8**). The osteotome should be sharp to allow easy division of the posterior scars and joint capsule. The authors prefer curved osteotomes. Curved osteotomes allow better entrance into the anatomically distorted subtalar joint. They serve as "prolongation of the surgeon's finger" and, by wiggling them within the subtalar joint, help to spread open the surgical area. The osteotome is inserted underneath the talar surface and passed down inferiorly and distally. One must make sure that the proper articular plane is hit (fluoroscopy). If the osteotome is found in the wrong plane, it needs to be removed and reinserted into the correct direction. This is an absolutely important step to get access for the later debridement of the posterior talocalcanear facets.

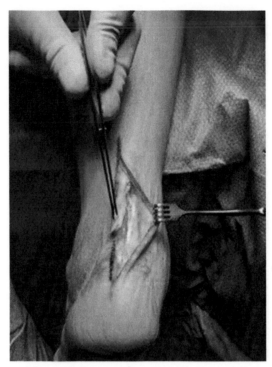

Fig. 6. The first step of the surgical procedure is to divide the Achilles tendon in a z-shaped way, which allows full access to Kager fat triangle.

A laminar spreader is inserted from the posterior into the subtalar joint (**Fig. 9**). Alternatively, a femoral distractor can be used. The advantage of the latter is that it does not block subtalar joint space. One pin is inserted into the calcaneal tuberosity, and a second pin is inserted in the distal tibia. Remaining cartilage and scar tissue are resected in their entirety using a slightly curved or straight rongeur.

The spreader and/or femoral distractor allow both opening of the subtalar joint space in order to adjust hindfoot height and accurate control of alignment. The surgeon must be careful not to set the hindfoot in varus or excessive valgus. The subchondral bone is perforated with a small drill or osteotome. The authors do not use burrs because of the heat developed by those instruments, which in turn may critically damage vascular supply of the bones.

Correction of hindfoot height is tested fluoroscopically (**Fig. 10**). Once completed, the void within the subtalar joint must be packed with structural bone graft (**Fig. 11**). Bone graft can be either allograft (eg, femoral head) or autograft (eg, posterior or anterior iliac crest). The shape of the bone graft needs to be formed according to need of hindfoot correction. Usually, the graft is trapezoidal in shape. When there is a varus hindfoot alignment present (most frequent deformity), the medial part of the subtalar joint needs to be elevated more to push the calcaneus into slight valgus and vice versa. The height of the bone block is selected according to the preoperative determination and amount of distraction needed to restore the hindfoot height. The final goal is to place the heel in neutral or slight valgus (ie, 5°). The authors use a push rod to impact the bone block into the subtalar joint. During impaction, it is mandatory to evaluate the alignment of the

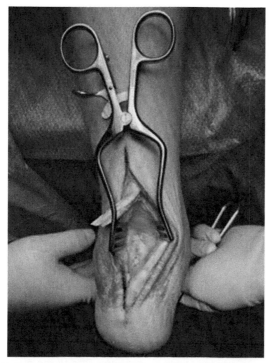

Fig. 7. The fat pad is incised and the subtalar joint reached. The capsule needs to be opened.

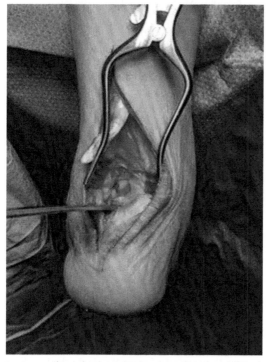

Fig. 8. Using an osteotome, the subtalar joint is opened and mobilized.

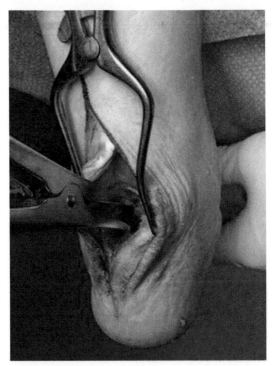

Fig. 9. After completion of subtalar joint mobilization, a laminar spreader is inserted to spread up the joint to the point where it should be corrected.

hindfoot. Besides clinical assessment of hindfoot alignment, fluoroscopy can be used to check the talocalcaneal angle and calcaneal axis (**Fig. 12**).

The final fixation is usually performed using one or 2 large screws entered from the plantar calcaneal tuberosity and extending into the talar body (**Figs. 13** and **14**). The principle applied is that of the so-called positioning screws. The authors most commonly use only one fully threaded 7.5-mm positioning screw to prevent postoperative collapse of the surgical construct.

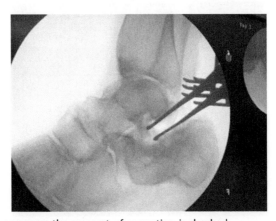

Fig. 10. Using fluoroscopy, the amount of correction is checked.

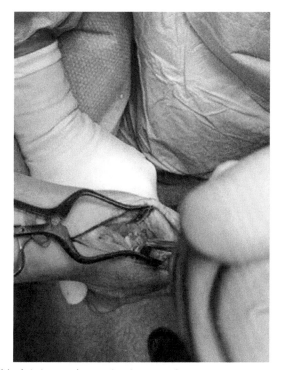

Fig. 11. A bone block is inserted to maintain correction.

Wound closure is performed by means of nonabsorbable 3-0 skin sutures.

Postoperative Regimen

The patient's leg is put in a plaster of Paris cast or a boot for 6 weeks postoperatively. Skin sutures are removed 2 weeks postoperatively. The patient is kept non-weight-bearing for a minimum of 6 weeks. Passive and actively assisted motions of the ankle and Chopart and Lisfranc joints can be commenced 3 weeks postoperatively.

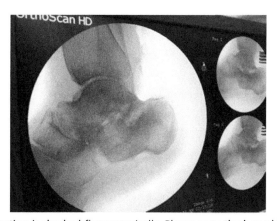

Fig. 12. The correction is checked fluoroscopically. Please note the bone block.

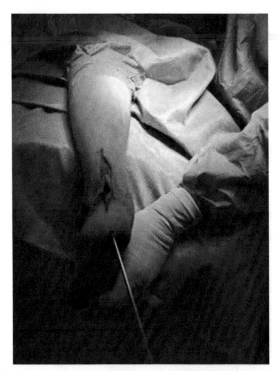

Fig. 13. The guide wire for the cannulated screws is inserted.

The authors require computed tomographic scans 6 weeks postoperatively to evaluate stage of union. Usually, patients need to be mobilized within the cast or boot for approximately 3 months. In the case of solid graft incorporation, the patient is gradually weaned off the boot or cast and begins with physical rehabilitation. Physical

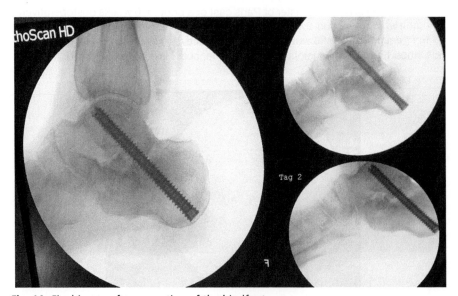

Fig. 14. Final image after correction of the hindfoot.

rehabilitation includes regaining calf strength, full mobilization of the ankle joint, and progressive proprioception.

PITFALLS AND POTENTIAL COMPLICATIONS

Nonunion is the most important complication of all.[13–15] In order to reduce the rate of nonunion, the authors have started to embed allograft bone into an autograft bone shell made up of cancellous bone. Autologous bone graft can be harvested from the posterior iliac crest. Alternatively, the autologous bone graft can be acquired from the distal tibia. When trying to harvest that kind of bone, the tibia should be exposed from strictly medially (5 cm proximal to the tip of the medial malleolus). A large curette helps to gather as much cancellous bone as possible.

By nature of the procedure itself, visibility of the surgical field is limited, especially when performing it through the posterior vertical approach. When there is no true option to visualize the surgical field properly, the authors almost always perform a z-shaped tenotomy of the Achilles tendon. By so doing, the tension is reduced and the visual field is enlarged, providing adequate size and access to operate on the subtalar joint. Alternatively, a surgeon might also use a straight lateral approach or the extensile approach to do a subtalar distraction arthrodesis. However, this decision must be made before starting the surgery (**Fig. 15**).

The sural nerve is at risk during this procedure. Direct trauma to the nerve by the approach or from traction after lengthening the hindfoot can cause significant damage. Therefore, the nerve should be identified and protected during the whole time of procedure.

Wound-healing problems are always a potential risk. To minimize that risk, the vertical posterolateral approach (as described in this article) is preferred. When augmenting the height of the hindfoot, increased tension on the skin will be the result. The vertical skin incision leads to approximation of the wound edges during tension, which facilitates closure.

Limited dorsiflexion at the ankle may not only be the result of a narrowed anterior ankle space but also a sequel of too much tension at the Achilles tendon. If there is

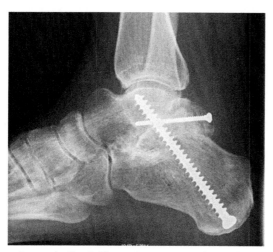

Fig. 15. The same patient as in **Fig. 1**. The postoperative radiographs reveal an elevation of the talus and strong fixation.

limited dorsiflexion of the ankle joint due to increased Achilles tendon pull, the authors almost always lengthen the tendon in a z-shaped manner.

Complications resulting from iliac crest bone graft harvest have been estimated up to 49%. Those complications include the risk of infection, residual pain (26%), and sensory loss.[16] Therefore, alternative sources of bone graft, that is, allograft, should be included in the decision making when embarking on surgery.

RESULTS

In 1988, Carr and colleagues[17] published their results of subtalar distraction arthrodesis in 16 patients after an average follow-up of 19 months. The union rate was 81%, and satisfactory results were achieved in 13 patients.

In contrast, Myerson and Quill[18] reported a union rate of 100% in 14 patients when using allograft bone. However, at time of follow-up (32 months), the results were only good in 50% of their patients (7 out of 14) and poor in 29%.

Bednarz and colleagues[15] performed subtalar distraction arthrodesis using iliac crest autografts. After a mean follow-up time of 33 months, the 64% of patients were able to return to either full- or part-time work. The union rate was 86%. The talocalcaneal angle and talar declination angle were significantly corrected. Almost all patients (96%) were satisfied after the procedure. In this study, 2 varus malunions (7%), 4 nonunions (14%), 1 metatarsal fracture (3%), and 1 plantar nerve paresthesia (3%) were found.

Shortly after Bednarz and colleagues, Burton and colleagues[19] published their own results of subtalar distraction arthrodesis in 13 cases after a mean follow-up time of 45 months. The union rate was 100%. The investigators found a significant improvement of the talocalcaneal and talar declination angles. Hindfoot height was changed by a mean value of 5 mm. Of all feet, 85% were rated as satisfactory.

In the study by Chen and colleagues,[20] 32 patients were evaluated for their results after subtalar distraction arthrodesis. The mean follow-up time was 71 months. Solid union was achieved in 97% of patients.

In 2001, Trnka and colleagues[14] reported on their results after subtalar distraction bone block arthrodesis. They included 39 patients (41 feet) who were treated by means of allograft and autograft bone blocks. Of those patients, 87% achieved full union. The final talar declination angle ranged 25° at time of follow-up. The mean increase of talocalcaneal height averaged 6 mm. Thirty-two fusions were considered successful, and 29 patients were satisfied.

Rammelt and coworkers[21] performed a subtalar distraction arthrodesis in 31 patients and reported a 100% union rate. Dynamic pedobarography revealed a return to normal with regard to pressure distribution during rollover and energetic gait.

Pollard and Schubert[13] investigated the results of 22 patients at a mean follow-up of 27 months. The mean increase of heel height was similar to all other studies (6 mm). The investigators found 1 nonunion, 1 subsidence of graft, 3 wound dehiscences, sural neuritis in 1 patient, painful hardware in 7 patients, and 1 mild varus malunion.

Garras and coworkers[22] studied the results of 22 patients at a mean follow-up of 36 months. In their study, 90% of cases achieved union. The mean time to union averaged 15 weeks. Two nonunions, 1 varus malunion, 1 sural neuralgia, and 1 case of bothering hardware were found.

More recently, Lee and Tallerico[23] presented the results of subtalar distraction arthrodesis in 15 patients (15 feet). Twelve frozen femoral head and 3 freeze-dried iliac crest allografts were used. After a mean follow-up time of 20 months, complete union was found in 93% of patients. The investigators added orthobiological agents to increase the rate of union. One nonunion was found. Eight minor complications were reported, including heel irritation (27%), 2 sural nerve paresthesias (13%), and 2 wound dehiscences (13%). The investigators concluded that the use of allograft was similar to autograft with regard to union and complication rates.

SUMMARY

In the presence of significant anatomic alteration at the level of the subtalar joint, it might be preferable to correct the position of the talus over the calcaneus and within the mortise. In order to estimate the amount of deformity, but also to get a better preparation in the preoperative setting, the talar declination angle is a very easy but helpful tool. It offers the option to define how much elevation should be needed to correct the talar location. A strictly posterior and longitudinal located approach provides good access to the subtalar joint. Elevation is best achieved by inserting a structural bone graft and securing with positioning screws. When respecting all the pitfalls of the procedure and performing adequate planning, the surgery can achieve very successful results.

REFERENCES

1. Gaul JS Jr, Greenberg BG. Calcaneus fractures involving the subtalar joint: a clinical and statistical survey of 98 cases. South Med J 1966;59(5):605–13.
2. Lapidus PW. Subtalar joint, its anatomy and mechanics. Bull Hosp Joint Dis 1955; 16(2):179–95.
3. Manter J. Movements of the subtalar and transverse tarsal joints. Anatomical Rec 1941;80(4):397–410.
4. Chandler JT, Bonar SK, Anderson RB, et al. Results of in situ subtalar arthrodesis for late sequelae of calcaneus fractures. Foot Ankle Int 1999;20(1):18–24.
5. Raymakers JT, Dekkers GH, Brink PR. Results after operative treatment of intraarticular calcaneal fractures with a minimum follow-up of 2 years. Injury 1998; 29(8):593–9.
6. Mulcahy DM, McCormack DM, Stephens MM. Intra-articular calcaneal fractures: effect of open reduction and internal fixation on the contact characteristics of the subtalar joint. Foot Ankle Int 1998;19(12):842–8.
7. Knupp M, Barg A, Bolliger L, et al. Reconstructive surgery for overcorrected clubfoot in adults. J Bone Joint Surg Am 2012;94(15):e1101–7.
8. Jahss MH. Evaluation of the cavus foot for orthopedic treatment. Clin Orthop Relat Res 1983;(181):52–63.
9. Huang PJ, Fu YC, Cheng YM, et al. Subtalar arthrodesis for late sequelae of calcaneal fractures: fusion in situ versus fusion with sliding corrective osteotomy. Foot Ankle Int 1999;20(3):166–70.
10. Myerson M. Reconstructive foot and ankle surgery. Philadelphia: Elsevier-Saunders; 2005.
11. Myerson M, Quill GE Jr. Late complications of fractures of the calcaneus. J Bone Joint Surg Am 1993;75(3):331–41.
12. Choudry UH, Bakri K, Moran SL, et al. The vascularized medial femoral condyle periosteal bone flap for the treatment of recalcitrant bony nonunions. Ann Plast Surg 2008;60(2):174–80.
13. Pollard JD, Schuberth JM. Posterior bone block distraction arthrodesis of the subtalar joint: a review of 22 cases. J Foot Ankle Surg 2008;47(3):191–8.
14. Trnka HJ, Easley ME, Lam PW, et al. Subtalar distraction bone block arthrodesis. J Bone Joint Surg Br 2001;83(6):849–54.

15. Bednarz PA, Beals TC, Manoli A 2nd. Subtalar distraction bone block fusion: an assessment of outcome. Foot Ankle Int 1997;18(12):785–91.
16. Ebraheim NA, Elgafy H, Xu R. Bone-graft harvesting from iliac and fibular donor sites: techniques and complications. J Am Acad Orthop Surg 2001;9(3):210–8.
17. Carr JB, Hansen ST, Benirschke SK. Subtalar distraction bone block fusion for late complications of os calcis fractures. Foot Ankle 1988;9(2):81–6.
18. Myerson MS, Quill G. Ankle arthrodesis. A comparison of an arthroscopic and an open method of treatment. Clin Orthop Relat Res 1991;(268):84–95.
19. Burton DC, Olney BW, Horton GA. Late results of subtalar distraction fusion. Foot Ankle Int 1998;19(4):197–202.
20. Chen YJ, Huang TJ, Hsu KY, et al. Subtalar distractional realignment arthrodesis with wedge bone grafting and lateral decompression for calcaneal malunion. J Trauma 1998;45(4):729–37.
21. Rammelt S, Grass R, Zawadski T, et al. Foot function after subtalar distraction bone-block arthrodesis. A prospective study. J Bone Joint Surg Br 2004;86(5): 659–68.
22. Garras DN, Santangelo JR, Wang DW, et al. Subtalar distraction arthrodesis using interpositional frozen structural allograft. Foot Ankle Int 2008;29(6):561–7.
23. Lee MS, Tallerico V. Distraction arthrodesis of the subtalar joint using allogeneic bone graft: a review of 15 cases. J Foot Ankle Surg 2010;49(4):369–74.

Moving?

Make sure your subscription moves with you!

To notify us of your new address, find your **Clinics Account Number** (located on your mailing label above your name), and contact customer service at:

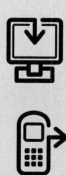

Email: journalscustomerservice-usa@elsevier.com

800-654-2452 (subscribers in the U.S. & Canada)
314-447-8871 (subscribers outside of the U.S. & Canada)

Fax number: 314-447-8029

Elsevier Health Sciences Division
Subscription Customer Service
3251 Riverport Lane
Maryland Heights, MO 63043

*To ensure uninterrupted delivery of your subscription, please notify us at least 4 weeks in advance of move.

Printed and bound by CPI Group (UK) Ltd, Croydon, CR0 4YY

08/05/2025

01864712-0001